M000017820

BEGIN
AGAIN
NOW

BEGIN AGAIN NOW
The Path to Fixing Health Care

Harry R. Jacobson, MD

Timothy C. Jacobson, PhD

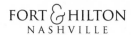
FORT & HILTON
NASHVILLE

FORT & HILTON
NASHVILLE

Copyright © 2016 by Fort & Hilton Publishing, Nashville, Tennessee

Printed and bound in the United States of America
Cover design: Gary Gore, Gary Gore Book Design
Typeset in Adobe Garamond and Quicksand
by Leann Davis Alspaugh | Orange Chrome

All rights reserved. No part of this publication may be reproduced,
stored in a retrieval system, or transmitted, in any form or by any means,
electronic, mechanical, photocopying, recording,
or otherwise, without the prior permission
of Fort & Hilton Publishing.

Library of Congress Cataloging-in-Publication Data
Begin Again Now: The Path to Fixing Health Care /
Harry R. Jacobson, MD, and Timothy C. Jacobson, PhD

pages cm
Includes bibliographical references.
ISBN 978-0-692-61713-7 (hardcover)

1. Medicine – United States – History. 2. Medicine – Policymaking –
United States – History. 3. Health care – delivery and regulation –
United States – History. 4. Flexner, Abraham – United States – History.
I. Jacobson, Harry R. II. Jacobson, Timothy C.

First Edition
5 4 3 2 1

*To future patients who will benefit
from the transformation
of health care delivery.*

CONTENTS

PREFACE

Where We Are and Why It Matters

American health care is on a dangerous course. There is wide agreement that our society can and should be healthier and that we should use less of our collective wealth in purchasing the health care required to achieve that goal. But costs are too high, while quality and outcomes are unacceptably low. That a system filled with brilliant, best-intentioned people is "dysfunctional" and in fact no system at all has become a sad front-page cliché for our times. Health care "reform," ever since creation of the Medicare and Medicaid entitlements in the 1960s, and as the *Stürm und Drang* surrounding Obamacare (officially—and perhaps ironically—the Affordable Care Act) reminds us, has focused historically on issues most attractive to the political classes and amenable, it has been thought, to engineering by legislative process: issues of access, coverage, and payment. The question of how we pay for health care and who receives it, however, has obscured the more fundamental question of what exactly it is we are buying. This is where American health care (and not, truth be told, America's alone) is on life support.

Current growth in health expense outpaces economic growth and is unsustainable, on its way from close to zero percent in 1970 to more than 20 percent of GDP in the near future. World Health Organization measures (World Health Statistics Part II: Global Health Indicators 2015) of the U.S. versus other countries do not make for happy reading. In health expenditures per capita in international dollars, the US ranks #1, France number #4, Canada #10 and the UK #26. For overall health-system performance, however, France is #1, the UK #18, Canada #30, the U.S. #37. Americans spend the most but take home the least. We spend more, critics say, because not everyone is uniformly insured and because we are allegedly less healthy than the rest of the developed world due to under-managed chronic diseases and unwise "lifestyle choices" (in other words, dubious tastes and risky habits).

But the real reason is simpler and less controversial: There is a huge gap between what we know and what we do, between the output of biomedical discovery and its translation into clinical practice and better health outcomes. This leads to crippling inefficiency in a delivery system beset by unlimited demand and insistent expectations, and to huge variability in cost and quality. Political efforts to control, regulate, and guarantee access miss this point and divert us from the root cause of this gap, which is structural and educational. This challenging state of affairs did not drop out of the blue. Nor is it attributable to villainous machinations of a once-imperious medical profession, or greedy insurance companies, or even meddling politicians and inept government bureaucrats. Rather, it is a consequence of history and the last big idea truly to reform American medicine, beginning a century ago.

This was an idea that put forward and then institutionalized the union of inductive science and clinical medicine, and that identified the physician-scientist as the prime mover in medicine's advance. The opening essay of *Begin Again Now* recounts the story of Abraham Flexner's famous reforms that so decisively accomplished this. It then follows Flexner's legacy into the clamorous junction between scientific medicine as he understood it, and the rise of health care as later generations redefined it. Flexner (1866–1959) was a man of his times, when expectations about what medicine could deliver were still modest, which is to say times rather different from now. Moreover, Flexner presumed that the service aspect of medicine—the way discovery made its way into the clinic and helped sick people—would more or less take care of itself. For a time it seemed to. But not forever, and as circumstances changed this critical presumption came unmoored from a system that, in our own day, delivers fragmented care and tolerates low quality.

The fundamental failure of the health-care service industry today (note that we avoid the phrase "health care system") is that it does not efficiently translate science into clinical practice. We do not understand now, and probably never will understand, all of medicine's mysteries, but we know for a certainty that we perform not nearly well enough with the knowledge we do have, and that realization grows daily clearer. This book makes a case for how to do better, not how to make things perfect. Great improvement is possible, even within our prevailing and self-limiting understanding of what medicine is and how it works. We grant, here at the beginning, that laboratory-orient-ed reductionist medicine as we have come to know it over the last century, with its fiercely instrumental worldview, is *not* all there is, and that the cause of beating back disease and improving health requires more than technology and improved understanding of molecular mechanisms although such tools re-main essential.[1] One of the most powerful orthodoxies of our time—the med-icalization of most human maladies—has not had the last word. It is however just this reductionist understanding of medicine, partial as it may be, that in our judgment is amenable to institutional renewal. The prescriptives described in this book along with a glance back at history may offer some guidance.

Flexner assumed that the translation of knowledge into practice would occur naturally, but he could not anticipate future execution challenges. Part of the challenge lies in how the health-care service industry is organized and how its workforce is educated and trained. It also results from how health-care services are paid for and who receives payment and for which services. The cur-rent "system" is based on physician autonomy whereas successful translation of science into clinical practice requires collaborative, integrated work teams that include physicians, nurses, pharmacists and other health professionals, plus patients and their families. In the current "system," physicians and in-stitutions feel they are accountable only for their own actions. The current "system" is literally disconnected, in that it fails to make the relevant infor-mation about the individual patient available to everyone who needs to know in order to make right decisions and deliver the right care. The current "sys-tem" does not leverage technology to increase its efficiency and effectiveness.

Bridging the gap between what we know and what we do today requires, then, another big idea, but a different one from Flexner's. It requires joining system to science as has not been done before, and it requires a new kind of doc-tor. The physician-scientists of Flexner's model are not about to disappear. But they will give precedence to physician-caregivers as the primary drivers down the road from discovery to improved health, and they will be joined by oth-ers. They will be men and women trained from the start to translate discovery, to use the evidence-base fully, to work in teams, to apply the power of infor-matics, and to improve their performance constantly and never stop learning.

The middle five chapters of *Begin Again Now* describe the components of this system. This is hardly fresh ground, any more than the union of inductive science and medicine was fresh with Flexner. But as then so now: It was by assembling and institutionalizing reform ideas in a new way that Flexner achieved broad and lasting impact. Therefore, even as we identify components of a new system of service, it is with the caveat that institutional arrangements once deemed optimum may no longer be so, and that the job of implementing a new system may require innovation here as well.

Flexner's original big idea—to cement the union of science and medicine by institutionalizing it in reformed medical schools—addressed problems of another era, namely, an oversupply of underwhelming medical schools and, consequently, a medical profession filled with too many doctors, too many of whom were substandard, and, consequently, with too many patients who were poorly served. Times change, and it should not surprise that solutions Flexner prescribed then—embedding medical schools in universities, a lockstep four-year undergraduate curriculum, the physician-scientist model, and so forth—have become problems now. But there is more to it than that. Flexner understood that his admittedly borrowed big reform idea, however virtuous its merits, could never capture medicine's commanding heights by scattershot assault alone. It required an executable plan of attack—a comprehensive order of battle. This remains as relevant as ever. Everybody knows what today's big ideas are, and, to repeat, our summary of them here is not offered as news. Rather, it is meant to help us focus on a model—a way of thinking about medicine and health-care service innovation—that, we believe, fits today's future just as Flexner's big idea fit yesterday's. There is no guarantee, of course, that this future will happen. We can however work to establish conditions that favor it.

If we are to close the gap between discovery and health outcomes today, then we must neglect neither these conditions nor Flexner's second great insight. He called it the Principle of Emulation whereby in medicine good drives out bad, and how a relatively small number of superior institutions can compel others to follow in their wake or fall by the wayside. Emulation explained how Flexner's program of disruptive reform achieved an impact disproportionate to the resources expended. Emulation, disruptive reform, and impact remain equally linked today. We conclude with practical proposals to "begin again now," by repurposing select existing institutions (and creating others *de novo*) whose measurable superiority will activate emulation and enable us at last to close the gap between what we know and what we do, between discovery and health.

HISTORY

Abraham Flexner's Dangerous Big Idea

Once upon a time, we called it the art of medicine. Then, we called it the science of medicine. Then, it became known as health care. Today, it is all a mess. Arguably no public policy issue of our times stirs more impassioned, often embittered, sometimes irrational debate than this one. How did it happen that the ancient art of healing as it evolved into the citadel of biomedical science came to occupy such contentious ground? Is it simply the price of success? Partly. To understand, it helps to recall the far history.

For millennia, medicine was random, haphazard, small-scale, often super-naturalist, largely ignorant of how our bodies work or sometimes fail to. Medicine cost little and was of small consequence to society. Before most physical and mental maladies, medicine's practitioners were impotent. Old-time doctors were satirized, not sued. Today, it's different. Medicine is massive, pervasively scientific and instrumental. It gives birth to great industries and costs measured in the trillions. It is of the greatest consequence to a society heavily invested in quality of life. Its practitioners enjoy power and prestige, yet they are embattled.

Medicine is about "health," but it is not the same thing as health. From ancient times until early in the twentieth century, medicine wrestled, without much success, with age-old challenges: to repair wounds, to ease pain, to cure sickness, to try to bring children into this world alive. But even as sound knowledge began to accumulate, starting in the Renaissance and continuing into the nineteenth century, little of it mattered to sick people. For them, medicine's long story was largely a tale of futility. And then, only about 100 years ago, the dam broke and things began to happen. The ascent of health, empowered by medicine, suddenly became possible. Medicine began to deliver more and more of the goods that it had long sought—and many it had never even imagined. And everyone wanted the goods.

In the first half of the twentieth century, Western medicine broke out or, to borrow a phrase from economics, it reached "take-off." This meant that medicine at last made the big leap between knowledge about how the body works and about the maladies that afflict it, and the ability of doctors (who more or less knew what they were doing) to beat back disease, heal the sick, extend life. At last, medicine found the pathway connecting cause to prevention and cure. And science has been the key.

It was an auspicious start, but what looked like a clear path then has become, in our own day, a crowded, congested, even crumbling highway. Science is better than ever, yet health remains elusive. While we know with some confidence *what* to do in order to bridge this gap—the gap between what we know and what we do, between discovery and health—we don't seem to be doing it broadly or consistently. What stands in the way? This book will argue that the problem relates back to a singular idea that has animated much of modern medicine's success story. This was how Abraham Flexner institutionalized the union of inductive science and clinical medicine in university medical centers and established the figure of the physician-scientist as prime mover in medicine's presumed perpetual advance. We also argue that embedded in the same idea can be found keys to solving today's puzzle. With medicine's long, largely dark history, this nearer period could not stand in sharper contrast, and it holds for us a double lesson—how past success can become, as time passes, a constraining legacy and yet preserve within it principles to guide action now.

Begin Again Now therefore both begins and ends with stories about the connection between transformative ideas and carrier-institutions. It begins in this chapter by recalling Flexner's story, the most recent epoch in medicine's modern history when a transformative idea and a particular class of institutions were, with stunning effectiveness, yoked together. The interior chapters of our book then move on to describe the big instrumental ideas of our own day: the *what* of what we need to do in order to bridge the gap from discovery to health. Our book concludes by returning to the subject of institutions and the question of how to institutionalize these transformative ideas as effectively now, as those were then.

Abraham Flexner: Brutally Frank Highwayman

On April 23, 1956, the American Medical Association (AMA), the Association of American Medical Colleges (AAMC), and the National Fund for Medical Education hosted a dinner in honor of Abraham Flexner and presented him with the Lahey Award for outstanding leadership in medical education. The award was named for Frank H. Lahey, Boston surgeon and founding trustee of the National Fund. The Fund had been established in 1949 under the titular leadership of Dwight Eisenhower, then-president of Columbia, former President Herbert Hoover, and James B. Conant, then-president of Harvard, and supported by the AMA, the AAMC, and others. Its purpose was to mobilize private support for the nation's medical schools and deflect the threat of government intrusion. The Fund was a fitting co-sponsor to honor Flexner, whose famous 1910 report calling for wholesale rebuilding of American medical education had triggered private benevolence on the unprecedented scale of $600 million–$700 million.

It was a formal affair at the Waldorf-Astoria in New York City, with a high and mighty guest list that included Dean Rusk, President of the Rockefeller Foundation, John W. Gardner, President of the Carnegie Corporation, Marion B. Folsom, Secretary of Health, Education and Welfare (standing in for Ike who sent a congratulatory letter), and the heads of fifty-seven of the country's eighty-one medical schools. The guest of honor, age 90, still sported his trademark pince-nez and, thanks to an honorary degree from Western Reserve University, shared the title of "Doctor" with the many others present.

Since publication of the Flexner Report in 1910, the Rockefeller philanthropies had taken the lead and done more than any other single source to fund the Flexner reforms. That spring evening in New York, Dean Rusk spoke the longest. Crediting his colleague John Gardner and the Carnegie Corporation for having started things off, he recalled how then-Carnegie president Henry S. Pritchett had "planted a seed in a wonderfully fertile spot, the mind of Abraham Flexner, and how that seed grew into *Bulletin Number Four* [*of the Carnegie Foundation for the Advancement of Teaching*]."[1] He spoke of Flexner's "brutal frankness" in assessing American medical schools in his survey forty-six years before and for his unapologetic "prejudice toward excellence." He spoke of the remarkable team of John D. Rockefeller, Jr. and Frederick T. Gates, who had read William Osler's *Principles and Practice of Medicine* in 1897 and drew conclusions that led to establishment in 1901 of the Rockefeller Institute for Medical Research, later headed by Flexner's older brother Simon. "Medicine can hardly hope to become a science," Rusk quoted Gates writing to Rockefeller, Sr., "until it can be endowed, and qualified men enabled to give themselves to uninterrupted study and investigation, on ample salary, entirely independent of practice." Rusk entertained guests with fragments of the 1911 conversation between Flexner and Gates that even then had entered the folklore of American medicine:

> Gates: "I have read your *Bulletin Number Four* from beginning to end. It is not only a criticism but a program.
> Flexner: "It was intended, Mr. Gates, to be both."
> Gates: "What would you do, if you had a million dollars with which to make a start in the work of reorganizing medical education?"
> Flexner: "I should give it to Dr. [William] Welch."
> Gates: "Why?"
> Flexner: "With an endowment of $400,000, Dr. Welch has created [at Johns Hopkins], in so far as it goes, the one ideal medical school in America. Think what he might do if he had a million more."

Rusk's listeners would have been familiar with rest of the story and indeed had lived through much of it themselves. Flexner soon joined the General Education Board of the Rockefeller Foundation and for the next fifteen years toiled successfully to realize much of what his report had recommended. Substantial grants went to key schools—Hopkins, Harvard, Yale, Chicago, Vanderbilt, Washington University, Tulane, Western Reserve, and Rochester—beacons to guide all others. Such exemplars would secure medical education as the responsibility of strong institutions of higher learning, governed by rigorous scientific discipline. Not even the Rockefellers could do it all, however, and Flexner soon became a familiar as well as a hard and persuasive bargainer with names like Rosenwald, Lasker, Whitney, and Morgan. George Eastman, not an easy touch, called Flexner "the worst highwayman that ever flitted into and out of Rochester. He put up a job on me and cleaned me out of a thundering lot of my hard-earned savings."

Rusk called special attention to Flexner's "principle of emulation," the way that in modern medicine good drives out bad. Leadership institutions, Flexner believed, raised the level of follower institutions that could ill afford to fall behind. In a famous example, the General Education Board made a large grant to the University of Iowa to reform its medical school, but Flexner flatly refused supplicants from neighboring states, saying "You will have to do it for yourselves. Our funds are not large enough." Then the twist of the knife: "You cannot afford to have it said in the Middle West that Iowa has something that your university lacks."

Before an audience of deans and administrators, Rusk spoke not primarily about history but about facing down problems, Flexner-style, as urgent in 1956 as in 1910. These same problems continue to demand our attention. Just as Flexner asked in 1910, we today could ask what to teach medical students within reasonable time limits, "out of the vast storehouse of advancing knowledge—a storehouse which defies a lifetime of learning?" How to bring that knowledge "to bear upon the patient when he turns to his doctor for help?" How to entice enough dedicated young people into careers in medicine to care for a rapidly growing population, and how to induce some to give their full time to teaching and research? How to maintain and expand "the intellectual capital that comes from pure or basic research … from which we draw the clues and solutions for practical problems?" How to retain contact with and "some human control over the flood of knowledge now flowing out of laboratories all over the world?" And of course, first and last, how to find the resources large enough to pay for it all?

Flexner's Report

Like the United States Constitution, the Flexner Report is a lodestone text, alternatively radical and conservative, innovative and owing much to precedent, subject to endless interpretation but difficult amendment. Both documents attempted, successfully, something very difficult. The Constitution was composed in the heat of crisis, begotten of hard compromise. Through it, multiple authors sought a formula for nationhood that would reconcile jealous and divided sovereignties. It established in broad stroke a federal union, leaving much of the detail for future generations to work out. In vagueness lay its genius. The Flexner Report was also composed at a moment of great urgency, of singular conviction but not compromise. It had just one author and laid out a future vision of medicine with breathtaking confidence. In certitude and right timing lay its genius. It detailed a template to institutionalize the union of science and medicine that was clear and, with money attached at the critical hour of creation, irresistible. For years, it carried all before it. A century later, the Flexner Report lives and breathes in every academic medical center in America and many around the world.

Between its publication and World War II, the report proved-out as few policy reports ever have, in the comprehensive re-making of American medical education. When Flexner spoke, men of means and action listened. For the first quarter of the twentieth century, along the closed corridors of the great foundations, in the universities and in the medical profession, Flexner, who was neither rich, nor an academic, nor a medical doctor, knew all the names and learned all the turnings. Whatever Flexner recommended happened.[2] At the time of the Waldorf-Astoria dinner, close to the end of a long life, the man who described as his personal motto "I burn that I may be of use," could look back with confidence that he *had* been.

Flexner's report was not original but consolidated and dramatically confirmed the work of others, who unlike himself, were medical men. In 1904, the American Medical Association established the Council on Medical Education as a central regulating agency in an attempt to raise standards in the profession and reduce the number of medical graduates. Led by Arthur Dean Bevan of Rush Medical College in Chicago, the council's five members (who included John A. Witherspoon from Vanderbilt) laid the groundwork for what ultimately became Flexner's report.[3] The council proposed its own improved standards for what a modern medical school should aspire to and suggested some minimum standards to apply immediately, such as a four-year course and requirement for a four-year high school education for admission. It even began its own inspection of the country's 160 schools in 1906 (five would close by the time of Flexner's visits). It ranked 82 as "acceptable," 78 as "doubtful" or no good at all. In 1908, at Bevan's bidding, Henry S. Pritchett, President of the Carnegie Foundation for the Advancement of Teaching allied Andrew Carnegie's philanthropy with the reform movement, agreeing to sponsor a second survey. This one was to be the work, deliberately, of a non-medical man and had the added aim of bringing the baleful state of medical education to the attention of those outside the profession.

What became *Bulletin Number Four of the Carnegie Foundation for the Advancement of Teaching*, the Flexner Report was both an American original and a catalyst that kindled change from ideas long lying about.[4] The story behind it is an oft-told tale, its enormous impact a compound of timing, luck, the skill of its author and the confluence of interests between an anxious profession and young philanthropies in search a winning cause. Flexner ascribed his own entrée into medical reform to his first book, *The American College*. Henry Pritchett had read and liked it and found in its author the ideal candidate to carry it out the Carnegie survey. Flexner was well-credentialed and came recommended by Ira Remsen, Daniel Coit Gilman's successor as president of John Hopkins, and by his brother Simon Flexner of the Rockefeller Institute, also a Hopkins-educated M.D. and bacteriologist. (Abraham had been in thrall to the Baltimore institution since his graduation from Hopkins in 1886 with an A.B.) Flexner accepted straightaway Pritchett's offer to tackle medical education head-on and, with a small salary but a large expense account, he set off in January 1909 on the whirlwind inspection of the country's 155 medical schools—the fieldwork for the report that would make him famous.

Flexner worked full-time and fast. In a year and a half, he was finished with his travels and his report. To generations of doctors since that time, it became axiomatic that Flexner's report marked the dividing line between the old medicine and the new. Because it recommended so much that in fact did come to pass and quickly, its iconic status as herald of a new era in medical education and in medicine was not surprising. From its forceful, fact-filled pages the future took shape.

The reality was not so discontinuous. As much meticulous documentation as fresh revelation, the report was a masterfully timed capstone to three decades of reform ideas as advanced by educators, scientists, and practitioners represented by a reinvigorated AMA and symbolized by the medical school of Johns Hopkins. But whereas reform up until Flexner had been halting and piecemeal, reform after Flexner accelerated and transformed into a national cause driven as much by laymen as by doctors, as much by institution-builders as by scientists. Pritchett, also a layman, understood this as the greatest barrier up to then. Writing in the preface to *Bulletin Number Four*, Pritchett observed: "The right education of public opinion is one of the problems of future medical education."[5] Flexner's polemic took on that challenge, and in doing so seized and held new ground. Flexner was convinced that reform, to succeed on the national scale that was called for, required both an argument sustainable beyond the medical community alone and a strategy capable of effecting institution-building. He supplied the argument; the foundations for which he soon became chief spokesman on this subject supplied the strategy.

He laid out afresh an argument that was at once both ancient and modern. It linked medicine (specifically, at that moment, medical education) to society's needs. Medicine's social mandate to attempt to heal the sick and do no harm went back millennia. But by Flexner's day, something new had entered the picture. Through the growth and improved application of scientific knowledge, the old art of medicine was improving fast and turning historic claims for healing into demonstrable clinical success. Although the antibiotic revolution that followed World War II would take place after Flexner had retired from the field, in the early years of the twentieth century while Flexner was hard at work, the new wisdom dictated that nothing worked in medicine quite like science. What had long been an art by default, ceased to be as bit by bit science began to unravel the mysteries of human biology.

Through hard work and careful clinical application, science in medicine kept a great many though not all of its promises. In the great era of reform that began with Flexner and for much of the century that followed, the science and the service of medicine seemed well joined. "The modern point of view may be restated as follows," Flexner put it characteristically without equivocation. "Medicine is a discipline, in which the effort is made to use knowledge procured in various scientific ways in order to effect certain practical ends."[6] (To say, as we would today, that the job of the health care service industry is to translate science into clinical practice expresses the same idea.)

Flexner factored into medicine's age-old social equation "the ideals of medical science." Then, as institutional innovator, he solved it in a way utterly hostile to the old-time proprietary medical schools that, in his view, had for so long oversupplied the country with underwhelming doctors. This was the startling programmatic heart of his report. His modern ideals were exotics that demanded special controlled conditions to flourish. What the country wanted was fewer but better medical schools producing fewer but better doctors. It was a radical, straightforwardly elitist proposition. Only the few were fit carriers for ideals, but the few must be trusted to serve the needs of the many. How many schools and doctors should there be? It was a key "social" question but not, incidentally, one unrelated to the high cost of reform and educating young doctors in the modern ways which tended naturally to limit their numbers. Precision about "the right number of doctors" was devilishly difficult then and now. (Flexner looked for guidance, as in so much, to German models.)[7] Whatever the exact sums might be, it was the logic that mattered. The quantities of medical graduates had to decline if science was to be advanced because only then would the medical needs of the country best be met. The procedure to accomplish this was simple: fewer and better doctors produced fewer and better doctors. Endowed, discriminating, and standardized medical schools of the reformed type were means to this end just as the old type of medical school—commercial, democratic, and idiosyncratic—were obstacles.

The particulars are well-known and became scripture: real admissions standards, a four-year course divided sequentially into preclinical and clinical subjects, teaching hospitals controlled by university administrations through full-time salaried faculty, organic university association, and insulation from the world of private practice. Everything served one high purpose: the practical application of scientific knowledge to the needs of the sick thus moving from bench and bedside.

Fixed and certain as the prescription seemed, it also presumed change. Medical education must continuously respond (at the moment Flexner wrote, catch up) to scientific discovery and social circumstances. Flexner never saw his work other than as the starting point of a long process. "The reconstruction [per *Bulletin Number Four*] of our medical education … is not going to end matters once and for all. It leaves untouched," he wrote with memorable phrasing, "certain outlying problems that will all the more surely come into focus when the professional training of the physician is once securely established on a scientific basis. At that moment, the social role of the physician will generally expand, and to support such expansion, he will crave a more liberal and disinterested educational experience."[8] A great deal of Flexner's prescription for reform proved extraordinarily lasting. It also proved just the opening gun in a race to keep medical education aligned with the growth of scientific knowledge and with the services that society expected of the profession. The race quickened as the "outlying problems" multiplied.

What Flexner Began

Between 1910 and century's end, more than a score of subsequent reports created a tradition of reform writing on medical education and the increasingly complex institutions where medical education—but not education alone—

occurred.[9] Titles bespoke the genre's earnest optimism—Planning for Medical Progress through Education, *A Handbook for Change*, *Healthy America: Practitioners for 2005*. In substance, virtually all displayed consistent central themes and together witnessed the tenacity of ideas in Flexner's original.[10]

In general, all of the subsequent reports partook of Flexner's social understanding of medicine and the medical profession—"The medical profession is a social organ, created not for the purpose of gratifying the inclinations or preferences of certain individuals, but as a means of promoting health, physical vigor, happiness and the economic independence and efficiency immediately connected with these factors"[11]—and the corollary that medical schools exist to serve society. The signature value remained Flexner's social status of medicine and the figure of physician as a "social instrument." "Medicine exists to serve society," and "must ever be responsive to the needs of the society it serves, said the AMA's *Graduate Education of Physicians* from 1966. Schools were producing too few "socially responsible doctors [who] recognize medicine as a social good, not a commercial commodity," echoed the Josiah Macy Foundation's *Clinical Education and the Doctor of Tomorrow* from 1989. Two years later, the Pew Health Professions Commission warned that the failure to respond better to the community of patients "violates the basic covenant between health professionals and the people they have obligated themselves to serve."

How exactly the schools served society of course changed over time. For the first decades after Flexner, training clinicians alone was seen to fulfill the obligation. By the 1950s, research took priority. "Research is an essential activity of any medical school," said the AMA's *Medical Schools in the United States at Mid-Century* from 1953. "It is the means whereby the schools seek to discharge their obligation for the advancement of knowledge." In 1982, the AMA's Council on Medical Education described the schools' frankly dual mission, as part of universities, both to educate students and generate fresh biomedical knowledge (*Future Directions for Medical Education*). Some reports specifically conjured the shadow of outside (government) regulation that awaited any learned profession that failed to reform itself and enforce standards of practice and education. From the AMA in 1966: "Responsibility can be assumed by society as a whole, operating through government, or can be assumed by the organized profession through a voluntarily accepted self-discipline." As demands for medicine's goods and services rose along with the advance of its knowledge, and as the environment for social entitlement expanded in the 1960s, the language describing medicines social nature also changed. "The number of those who make demands upon the medical profession has steadily increased," from the American Surgical Association in 1966. "But superimposed upon this increase in numbers has been an ever more significant increase in expectations." (*Medical Education Reconsidered*) And from the AMA in 1982: "Expectations have not been realistic."

Beneath the medicine-as-service umbrella, post-Flexner reports asked similar questions about the future and finding the way ahead. What precisely does it mean to serve the public interest? How to calibrate the tricky ratio of physician supply to the size and needs of the population? How to contain, manage, and translate the explosion of medical knowledge? How to modulate the bias for clinical specialism and reemphasize generalist education?

On how better to serve the public interest, the 1932 report of the American Association of Medical Colleges (AAMC), *Medical Education: Final Report of the Commission on Medical Education*, echoed Flexner without embellishment on the importance of achieving closer alignment with the needs of society. Sixty years later the Pew report, *Health Professions Education for the Future: Schools in Service to the Nation* (1993), turned up the volume considerably, speaking of "this most human of all enterprises—welcoming new life, aiding the sick, comforting the dying" and warning that only reassertion of "the fundamental values that define and shape their calling" could keep the medical profession from devolving into "associations for health care workers."

The second question, about workforce issues and how society could secure the right number of doctors, took on fresh urgency starting in the mid-1960s, when improvement in medical education came to be equated with more medical graduates. From the AAMC's 1965 report *Planning for Medical Progress Through Education*: "Most [persons] point to the need to take major steps to improve medical education—to enable the nation to produce more and better prepared physicians and other health personnel."

On the third question, of how to deal with ever more information, the same report fretted that "the phenomenal growth of knowledge has increased at an ever-accelerating pace." And although schools still attempted it, "it is becoming more and more apparent to the educator that it is no longer possible to provide encyclopedic coverage of the contents and skills of medicine within the limited time available." In 1992, the Robert Wood Johnson Foundation report,

Medical Education in Transition warned of an information load "to strain human cognitive capacities" and that, in the future, management not mastery of information would be the critical factor in any effective system of medical education.

The fourth question, about excessive specialism and the temptation to allow fields of practice shape the medical school curriculum, also yielded consistent response. "Changes in the methods and forms of practice should not," asserted a 1932 AAMC report, "be the guide for determining the educational needs of medical students." In 1989, the report of the New York Academy of Medicine, *The Graduate Education of Physicians*, lamented the drift of clinical education away from "a broad preparation of the undifferentiated doctor" toward "an increasingly fragmented, technically-oriented training program for specialists."

The tradition of reform confirmed the introspectiveness that Flexner bequeathed to medical education, and not to education alone. The regular appearance of sequels to his report and the consistency of their content also raised a question.[12] Was medical education somehow intrinsically substandard and thus perpetually in need of fixing-up? Indeed, did medicine as a whole? Would we, could we ever get it right? Did endless calls for reform in presence of, some said, little real change, constitute a fool's errand?

In truth, medical education was probably no more resistant to improvement than other forms of schooling. It was suggested, in reality, that the tradition of reform reports following from Flexner could be accounted for by purposes tangential to education but directly related to the larger subject of medicine and health. According to this argument, the post-Flexner reports served largely to reaffirm "certain core values of the profession" and to legitimate its continuing self-regulation.[13] Others went further to suggest that such a long history of "reform without change" could only be accounted for by the unfruitful competition between education and research where education always lost out: "Medical education's manifest humanistic mission is little more than a screen for the research mission."[14] An overstatement perhaps, but as medical schools evolved into the modern medical centers, it was natural that invocations to reform should reach beyond purely educational realms to address burgeoning research and patient care enterprises.

Beyond dispute, the stream of reform reports revealed just how effectively that first one, not yet again equaled, had done its work. Flexner's polemic and the philanthropic muscle that backed it up made change happen. Medical schools became firmly rooted in universities, mostly in medium and large-sized cities. Admission requirements and curricula were reformed, as he said they must be. Four-year graded courses became universal. Faculties and their hospitals became dedicated to teaching, not practice. Commercial schools closed. Flexner's famous maps (see chapter six) depicting his proposal for the reduction and geographical distribution of medical schools have been followed reasonably well. Scientific medicine pushed medical sects beyond the pale of respectability and out of competition. State regulatory bodies and boards of medical examiners enforced higher more exclusive professional standards. Postgraduate work ceased in its old role as undergraduate repair shop to become an intensive, highly specialized activity within the university system.

It was a broad victory though not without irony. Flexner helped achieve standardization in general medical education just as the practice of medicine, in both private practice and university teaching settings, was, thanks to science, growing more specialized. This in turn threatened the alliance of interest between practitioners and academic doctors that had united them behind reform in the first place. The new system was calibrated to create one kind of doctor for many different needs, while there were those who said that the realities of practice demanded something else. Nor did all who posed as his disciples in years hence see in it quite the same unity that Flexner did. They tended to fall into two groups. To many academic doctors and probably to most doctors in private practice in the United States, *Bulletin Number Four* was the fountainhead for the doctrine of scientific excellence, personified in the figure of the physician-scientist. They could point to its emphasis on training in the basic sciences and mastery of the scientific method, and they embraced clinical training in university teaching hospitals where young apprentices learned by doing under the eye of watchful masters. Others, while not dissenting from the doctrine of scientific excellence, re-emphasized Flexner's other message about medicine's social function, one that the chorus of scientific excellence threatened to drown out. What would become, they asked, of Flexner's concern for matters of preventive medicine, public health, and broadly speaking, public service? Once the knowledge was secured, how then to deliver the service?

After Flexner

It is important to trace the history a bit further. Flexner's famous reforms were clearly conceived and boldly executed. They were all brilliant. They all worked. And eventually they stopped working. Three connected factors—the fruits of discovery, health care and rights, and finally, the cost of it all—explain why. At first, science truly did bear fruit, and medicine picked off the easy bits quickly and effectively. But along with new science-enabled clinical success came rising expectations about health, which was increasingly seen as medicine's product. Accompanying rising expectations were implication and then assertion of the right to health care and the useful service that medicine now made possible. The more people assumed that they were entitled to health care (what had once been known as medical care) along with the products and technologies that enabled it, the more creative became public and private responses to satisfy, painlessly at first, that limitless demand. Enter third parties and the progressive insulation of consumers from costs.

The Fruits of Discovery The purpose of medicine is to serve, of science to know, and the coming together of helpful service and useful knowledge took some time. The first great successes of research came in the field of infectious diseases, beginning in the 1930s with the development of penicillin and in the 1940s and 1950s of other chemotherapeutic agents that attacked the specific microbial agents known to be fundamental mechanisms of disease. Wartime accelerated research and development more quickly than at any time in its long past. Medicine grew measurably better at what it had long claimed to be able to do. With the "antibiotic revolution" of the early postwar years, once largely untreatable bacterial infections like pneumonia, tuberculosis, syphilis, polio, and typhoid came under medicine's effective control.

Scientific and clinical advance occurred against a policy background that was destined to cast a long shadow, as private insurance regimes developed to spread risk and ensure access to medicine's bounty across the general population. As science proved its therapeutic value, and as the presumption of uniformly high quality settled in, the central challenge became one of how to socialize the costs of modern medicine. Who paid and who received access?

The rise of broad-based group health insurance in the United States dates to the founding between the world wars of Blue Cross: insurance plans that paid for treatment in hospitals on a cost-plus (cost of service plus cost of capital) basis. When price controls during World War II prevented wage competition for scarce labor, many firms embraced fringe benefits including hospital and health insurance, the cost of which in 1943 became tax-deductible for businesses, while the benefits became tax-exempt for workers. In the postwar years, the system of employer-based insurance grew broadly and benignly, dominated by nonprofit organizations, which operated on the principle of community rating (equal premiums regardless of risk) and pooling (whereby high and low risk individuals bought coverage together). If the pool was large enough, the result was a kind of social insurance based on membership in the group, and not on need for service. By the late 1970s, 85 percent of American civilians were covered by such an employer-based private system.[15]

Health Care and Rights   Medicine cannot escape its social, cultural, and economic contexts, so it was not well-prepared for the tumult of the 1960s and 1970s. At first, when times were good and national self-confidence high, the names our leaders gave to those years—the New Frontier and the Great Society—served to mobilize popular idealism and reconfirm, it seemed, institutionalized national meanings. The peculiarly American ambition to do all things well for all people all of the time boldly asserted itself. Medicine, which in previous decades had so well proven its promise, seemed an easy target. And this was when the language changed. Medicine ceased to be "medicine" at all and became "health care." The World Health Organization's expansive 1946 definition of health as "a state of complete physical, mental and social well-being and not merely the absence of disease or infirmity" set the tone, and the words mattered. Medicine was precise and limited; health care was something else, altogether more comprehensive. In addition to the biological factors that were the domain of scientific medicine, health care, we soon learned, encompassed social, economic, environmental, and spiritual factors. Not only were traditional providers looked to for medicine, they were also relied on for health—a mandate altogether more extensive than any that had come before.

The right to health care and by implication even to health itself became explicit, in the United States, with the entitlement reforms of the 1960s that created Medicare and Medicaid.[16] Accordingly, the conversation changed. More and more, Americans assumed they were entitled to medical or health care along with the products and technologies that enhanced it. To satisfy such a right in a society of finite productive capacity could of course require giving to some while disadvantaging others. Evolving systems of health care provision reflected such anxieties.

In post–World War II America, a good job meant one that offered not only good pay and some security but also health insurance. For those outside the employment-based insurance system, a net of public health coverage addressed the same expectation. The Hill-Burton Act of 1946 conditioned public subsidy for hospital construction on the provision of free care for the uninsured poor. In 1965, landmark federal legislation created Medicare and Medicaid, entitling the elderly and the poor to medical coverage. Both public and private insurance systems paid providers on the principle of "usual and customary charges," a notion rooted in a pre-insurance era when the fees that physicians could charge for service were subject to price competition. Third-party payment through insurance, however, desensitized patients to price and even upended classical economic behavior, as price often came to be correlated with quality. As long as the definition of "usual and customary" remained whatever the market would bear, costs rose even as new technology spread, which in other industries would have driven costs down. Meanwhile, for-profit insurers offering lower risk-rated premiums to attract healthier people began to punch big holes in the Blues' pool.

The Cost of It All   The entitlement reforms of the 1960s may have advanced social justice, but they failed to address cost. As an aging population suffering more from chronic maladies than from infectious diseases spiked demand for health care services, the cost of provision approached levels that threatened to overwhelm other national priorities. By the 1980s, the distress of America's once virtuous, parallel private/public system had grown acute, resulting in calls for "reform" across the political spectrum. Efforts to control costs were less than successful. In 1983, Medicare, which set the pattern for private insurers as well, attacked the cost-plus principle for hospitals with its Inpatient Prospective Payment System based on Diagnosis Related Groups (DRGs). While DRGs reimbursed fixed fees based on diagnosis, prospective payment stopped short of relating payment to results, and while hospital stays indeed went down, quality could go down too due to perverse incentives to under-treat. Physicians' fees came under this imperfect prospective payment regime in the 1990s, as did outpatient hospital care in 2000.

Accuracy of Cost Predictions

ESTIMATE	ACTUAL
1965 House Ways & Means "By 1990 Medicare A would be $9 billion"	$67 billion
1967 House Ways & Means "Total Medicare by 1990 would be $12 billion"	$110 billion

Source: Health Care Investment Group slide.

The subsequent movement to "managed care" bet on competition among insurers to drive costs down and on oversight of care by primary care physicians. More new phrases soon crowded the industry glossary, as Health Maintenance Organizations and Preferred Provider Organizations stepped in to negotiate prices with providers and, as it turned out, to manage (and micromanage) physicians. Capitation schemes (which paid fixed fees per enrollee per time period and allowed providers to keep the change if care turned out to cost less than the fee) further buttressed incentives to reduce costs and, like DRGs, cut down hospital stays. To maintain prices and margins, providers predictably pushed back against large health plans and zealous managed care administrators, consolidating and investing, sometimes redundantly, in facilities and technology. Reform reached near-fever pitch in the failed 1993 plan of the first Clinton administration, which proposed to insure the uninsured, oversee pricing nationally, and organize Americans into health insurance purchasing cooperatives. The debate continued to center on costs and access, leaving assumptions about quality still largely undisturbed.

Some two decades later the Affordable Care Act (ACA) of 2010, popularly loved or loathed as "Obamacare," after the president who made it his great cause, played on many of the same themes and re-jigged the old pieces (and some new ones) into legislation of daunting complexity and intense partisan flavor. The ACA was the largest expansion of the government entitlement to health care since the original Medicare and Medicaid legislation of the 1960s, but unlike those landmark reforms it became law without Republican support and was destined for rocky implementation and indeterminate outcome. The law was the most radical expression to date of a longstanding egalitarian impulse in American life as applied to the provision of health care, specifically the conviction that health care is a positive right to which all citizens must be assured equal access. The ACA did not turn America into a single-payer system, as many on the left had hoped, and probably still do hope. Nor was it strictly speaking "socialized medicine," as many on the right characterized it. Rather it subsidized, and forced into the regime of private insurance, several millions of Americans who for one reason or another (pick one: poverty, improvidence, simply choosing not to insure?) had been outside it before and presumably, therefore, were less healthy. It ratcheted-up aggregate demand without bothering much about shortfalls in supply. The goal to bring better care at lower prices to everyone remains afar off. For its fiercest partisans, however, the ACA at least achieved a step forward for social justice: the right thing to do even if it was not, at first anyway, particularly well-done.[17] What follows in the chapters to come is no further critique of such history, which is still in the making. Rather it is a look around us, and ahead of us, at the instrumentalities—translating discovery, using the evidence-base, working in teams, applying the power of informatics, constantly improving performance—that shift the focus away from who pays and who gets paid and onto what it is we all are buying. For make no mistake, whether or not it is a right, health care is a highly-desired and costly service, whose price would in other industries focus fierce attention on the best value for money. As for how to institutionalize value in health care, as Flexner institutionalized science in medicine, we are still only at the beginning of the story.

ONE

Translating Discovery

What is biomedical research worth? History suggests that its value in the past has been enormous. To modern secular cultures, which place premium value on physical health and long life, improvements in longevity obviously have advanced the general welfare and continue to do so.[1] Before the middle of the twentieth century, it was improved measures in public health and general economic development that mostly delivered the valued goods.[2] Since then, the fertile union of science and medicine carries the good work forward, with gains in health chiefly attributable to the decline in mortality among the middle-aged and elderly from cardiovascular disease and improved treatment of heart attacks thanks to medical research. Enthusiasm for scientific advance into the understanding of disease mechanisms, and the development of therapies that reliably work, suggest that for all that America spends on research, perhaps we should spend even more. Improved longevity contributes to economic growth and national wealth at levels, since 1950, equaling all other forms of consumption combined.[3] It is calculated that if mortality from cardiovascular disease and cancer were to fall just 10 percent, GDP would raise $10 *trillion.*[4] We know that the allegedly stratospheric costs of FDA-approved new drugs are relative, and that in fact the economic benefits far exceed them.[5]

We are less certain about how much "better health" is to be gained by increases in research (or care) expenditures at the margin. America spends vastly more per capita on medical research than the nations of the European Union.[6] In 2012, total US biomedical research and development expenditures (public and private) were only slightly less than the totals for Europe, Japan and China combined.[7]

Whatever understanding of disease processes that this commitment of resources may have bought (and it has bought a great deal), it has not secured, relative to other developed but notably more penurious nations, better health outcomes.[8] High research expenditure and stagnating health outcomes would seem to point toward pervasive challenges in the system (or lack of system) of care delivery, which is where debate on health care reform should land. It is a mistake however to lose sight of the prior challenge, of clarifying the processes connecting research to the point where delivery can begin and impact be felt.

Public and Private Biomedical Research and Development, 2007–2012 (US$ billions)

REGION	2007	2010	2012
United States	131	126	119
Europe	84	81	82
Asia/Oceana	41	53	62
Japan	28	35	37
China	2	4	8

Source: *New England Journal of Medicine*, January 2, 2014.

Translation Remembered

Pick any academic health center today, or any pharmaceutical or device or biotech company worldwide, and you will hear the buzzword "translation." This was not always so. Twenty-five years ago, while the concepts and indeed the practice of translation were hardly unknown, the word in the vernacular of that era referred less to something that happened in laboratories and clinics than in classics and modern language departments. The parallels are instructive. Language translation requires, first, a grasp of the fundamental difference between two different modes of expression, followed by the discovery in practice of how another language is built not of words in isolation but of structures and patterns that constitute grammar, syntax, and idiom. Even as they are codified in rules, the structures of language are dynamic, constantly re-shaped by use and culture. We understand this instinctively with our native tongues but commonly must learn it afresh for foreign ones, at least in our first encounters, if we wish to translate successfully. We recall the shock of this discovery in a first Latin class, finding ourselves suddenly at sea among declensions and conjugations, the mysterious and subtle signals conveyed in word endings and the strange (to an English-speaker's eye) placement of parts of speech.

It quickly becomes clear that translation is no rote dictionary exercise but hard intellectual work. Given a good teacher, we slowly acquire the tools and begin to get the hang of it; we learn to work through the obstacles and barriers and achieve results. And then, as if in discovery, we have something: a page of Cicero in English that represents the original Latin. Not literally of course. Sometimes little, sometimes much that is of cultural, historical, or poetic importance can be "lost in translation." The two versions of Cicero can never be identical. But meanings can be made clear: things make sense, and our understanding is advanced. Or, foreign languages aside, we have all experienced the frustration of attending to the speaker or writer who is over-fond of jargon or techno-speak, and to whom the only response is a "please, could you translate that for me into plain language?"

The plain language of medicine is, or ought to be, effective service to patients and improved health status of populations. The "translation" necessary to express this language means moving knowledge from basic science through clinical medicine to better health care. It is a challenge equal to mastering Latin. The obstacles inherent in all medicine—variation, uncertainty, and scarcity—abound.[9] The avenues of translation increasingly are not pure but mixed—private and public, academic and corporate, through all of which swirl an ever-changing diversity of people, processes and technology.

Applying the word "translation" to the movement of knowledge from basic science to better health conveys a sense of urgency that is new—the realization that this is something that will not happen on its own or at least not happen fast enough to satisfy current acute demand. During the 1950s, the phrase "simultaneous translation" came into common use in another context, referring to the need of diplomats at the United Nations to understand one another's speeches more or less as they were spoken or, as we might say today, "in real time."[10] The job market boomed for quick-thinking and quick-tongued interpreters who could manage, often hour after hour, to deliver both words and meanings with unfailing speed and accuracy. While this may be too much to hope for in science, medicine and health care, somehow translation must be speeded-up. There are ways to begin now.

Translation Restored

It would appear there is cause to worry. Over the past decade, and despite advances in molecular biology and identification of new therapeutic targets from the human genome project, the approval of new drugs has declined. Nine out of every ten new drug candidates fail regulatory approval and commercial development, and the one that succeeds takes a decade to develop and totes up a daunting investment price tag of $1 billion.[11] From the pharmaceutical industry perspective, drug development is hugely expensive and fraught with risk, and the challenges seem endless. The easy diseases have already been tackled, and novel therapies grow harder to conjure. Clinical trials, the last step in research and translation process, grow more complex and demanding, of patients, time and money. The biotechnology industry, second in hyperbole only to the advent of computers some twenty-five years prior, in fact has turned in a lackluster performance.[12] The general sluggishness in turn spurs political anxiety over how well public funds for academic research are being spent and why the clinical benefits, measured ultimately in health outcomes, are not more evident.[13]

History suggests that modes of translation, and the ways translation has been attempted, vary with the tools available to do the job.[14] From the 1920s through the 1950s, the golden age of the Flexner model for institutionalizing the union of science and medicine, discovery of new insights into human biology applicable to specific disease challenges arose, very largely in the Osler tradition, from careful clinical observation. It was an era when maladies typically presented late in their natural history and when therapies still were few. Crude measurement tools, expensive assays, and still modest physiological and biological understanding hampered basic science investigators in making connections with biomedical research at the clinical level. The notable successes of those years rested more on keen bedside observation than laboratory prowess; one thinks of Fuller Albright's work in endocrinology at Massachusetts General Hospital and his namesake clinical syndromes, or Alfred Blalock's studies at Vanderbilt and then Johns Hopkins on shock and "blue babies." With the burst of innovation in biochemistry and the advent of molecular biology that began in the 1960s, the balance tipped back the other way, and the path of translation opened up impressively, moving from basic science outward to the clinic. Better science plus keener tools and methodologies for applying science beyond the laboratory bench created fresh opportunities for clinical investigation at the bedside. The vagueness with which basic science could target clinical problems, however, remained an obstacle that would be overcome only—but then resoundingly—with the progress of genomics and proteomics at the end of the twentieth century. The Human Genome Project at last put key pathways and genetic agents of complex but widespread genetic disorders of the sort that consumed inordinate health care resources inefficiently, squarely within the cross hairs of basic science. When that happened, Flexner's old presumption about the natural transfer of scientific understanding of human biology into medical practice gained new life. Moreover, this fresh new potential to overcome the old barriers between science and medicine by using real patients with target diseases as models for identifying proteins and genes underlying them was characterized by a dynamic, back-and-forth process. This was in contrast to earlier modes of translation marked, if successful, by one-way linear progression. The mechanics of translation henceforth would not be the primary problem. While the science would never be complete, enough of it was done to render the largest obstacles to efficient translation less technical than organizational, political, and economic.

The first, and as of this writing, the only textbook on the subject of clinical and translational science begins with a telling disclaimer that, just as this is a field where Charles Darwin left an early imprint, it is subject today to "considerable evolutionary pressure." And it urges an inclusive definition of translation—"projection of proof of concept in cells and model systems into studies designed to elucidate human physiology or drug action"—to attract physician- and non-physician scientists alike and so do away with the division between pre-clinical "basic science" research and clinical research.[15] Indeed, Darwin, Claude Bernard, and Gregor Mendel laid the foundations of modern clinical and translational research in the nineteenth century before there ever was such a divide, and the infrastructures, both academic and industrial, that promise to bring it to fruition in the twenty-first century further deconstruct the old boundaries and point to translation as a relentlessly interdisciplinary challenge.[16]

Responsibility for clinical and translational research in the United States has resided historically within the realm of the academic health centers (AHCs) that evolved from the reformed medical schools of the pre–World War II era. There, the science of deliberate patient-oriented research began to take on institutional form and to prove its worth. This did not occur however at any scale without support external to the AHCs. Through the 1950s and 1960s, research-oriented AHCs had come to rely on the National Institutes of Health (NIH) as their primary pillar for research support, accepting its high scientific standards but also, albeit at arm's length, placing themselves within the orbit of expectations surrounding a publicly-funded federal agency. Translational research specifically found an academic home in NIH-funded General Clinical Research Centers (GCRCs), a program eventually spread across some seventy-five of the nation's research-oriented AHCs.[17] There, clinical investigators experienced the encouragement of collaborative research rare in ordinary academic settings and profited from the presence of critical intellectual mass.[18]

Diversity and integration of talent, from MD and PhD scientists to nurses and technicians, development of core laboratories, and a clear sense of mission all set GCRCs apart within busy workaday hospital settings, providing the controlled environment necessary for doing good science with a focus on patients. The results were gratifying, but as science changed, particularly as understanding of the genome increased and new instrumentation brought greater precision to investigative techniques, demands increased as well. New understanding of environmental factors in health and disease further expanded the scope of fresh opportunities, but not necessarily that of new resources. And while the clinical science amassed by the GCRCs was impressive within its realm, the connection to improved health status more broadly was still, to many, less convincing. In the context of accelerating scientific discovery and heated anxiety over what it all meant, experts posited different levels of obstacles to more effective translation of science into health. First obstacles occurred between initial discovery, either in the lab or at the bedside, and the next stage of clinical investigation. A second level occurred between proof of efficacy in human research and actual clinical practice. A third bottleneck referenced application to practice broadly and among large populations.[19]

Evidence that the blockages were real could be read in the famine-amidst-plenty phenomenon that from the late 1990s and into the new century beset the pharmaceutical and biotech industries referenced above. Never before had there been such technology with the potential to speed the translation process—from DNA databanks linked to de-identified electronic medical records to revolutionary imaging technology—and yet the pace of FDA approval of new molecular entities mired to a crawl. Were AHCs doing their part in clinical research? Was industry contributing? Was government helping or hindering the process? What were the ways to improve, or indeed to establish, the linkages among public and private, academic and commercial entities in the profession, and in the business, of translation?

One attempt to address the problem of improving the interaction between AHCs and the private sector was the establishment in 2005 of the NIH's Clinical and Translational Science Award (CTSA) program as successor to the GCRCs.[20] The program is still very young and the only definitive judgment thus far is that the ambition of the mandate surpasses the level of funding. Even so, the CTSA program represents a fresh approach to a newly urgent, old problem. As individual research institutions wrestled with creaky administrative structures and ways of thinking, it became apparent early that no single CTSA was likely on its own to punch through the obstacles to more efficient translation and that a consortium approach would be necessary. The initial goal was to implement sixty CTSA programs by 2012, which was accomplished, all resting on the founding conviction that translational research is a special discipline that, in order to thrive efficiently, needs an academic home and protected environment other than the traditional subject-limited academic department. To achieve the mission that flowed from it—"to transform the local, regional, and national environment to facilitate clinical and translational science, thereby increasing the efficiency, quality, and speed of clinical research"—required the sustained presence of faculty in multiple disciplines and attention to the kinds of patient-oriented research that would attract and retain the best talent into training and then careers in the discrete discipline of translational science.[21] It soon became apparent that one of the areas calling for cooperative approaches among the consortium of CTSAs would be transcending local issues. Such an issue was the matter of clinical research management systems, which analyzed typically insufficient informatics capabilities in order to find more fruitful forms of interface between informatics and improved management. Building up a national research inventory was another priority, aiming to identify the greatest capabilities of individual programs and link them via interoperable information technology. Informatics capabilities also pointed to the creation of a national clinical data system to render more compatible the data criteria employed in different institutions and projects, while a model for community engagement replicable at a national scale was deemed necessary to encourage community participation in clinical research and to find ways to focus on the problem of health disparities. Finally, there was need, across CTSAs, for a career support system or ladder, a training component that would ensure a fresh stream of young talent coming into the programs, and, in addition, build bridges between basic scientists and clinical investigators.[22]

All were very much works in progress, and future development no doubt promised shifts in emphasis and new initiatives, as some challenges yielded to early improvement while others proved more stubborn.[23] What the CTSAs did make unquestionably clear at the outset—and an insight that the future would only sharpen—was that clinical and translational research was the ultimate expression of team science and team medicine. It was an insight about how to achieve and sustain better connectivity between the two classical halves of the Flexnerian model of education and research. It demanded collaboration and partnerships and foreswore scientific fame and fierce clinical autonomy. Beneath its administrative cumbersomeness (at the beginning at least), the CTSAs represented a radical attempt to institutionalize and thus sustain translation at a new level of efficiency. The legacy research institutions of basic science and clinical care (chiefly AHCs) were designated the initial carriers of this culture—namely, Duke University, one of the most prestigious, received one of the very first CTSA awards and has since maintained a leading place in clinical and translational research.[24] Other organizational forms, if not yet common, are possible—namely, the Scripps Translational Science Institute founded in 2006 by Scripps Health System and thus far the only member of the CTSA consortium not affiliated with a university.[25]

The Use of It All

Discussion of translational science and research, and how both to institutionalize and accelerate it, belongs within the context of the shifting understanding of the connections between basic research, technological innovation, and social utility more generally, since World War II. What was once almost blithely deemed a linear process, flowing from basic research through to development and industrial application and, presumably, on to social utility, is now known to be otherwise. The pathways between scientific and technological innovation, in Donald Stokes's words, are "multiple and complex and unequally spaced."[26] Far from a smooth current, movement among them is frequently choppy and not immune to deep turbulence. Sometimes it even appears to flow in reverse, as technology inspires science rather than the other way around. Moreover, ultimate practical applications of technological innovation are not always as initially imagined. Steam engines were at first put to work pumping water from mines, but then adapted to make possible the transportation revolution that was the railroad. Radio, far more than just a "wireless" substitute for telegraphy, spawned a new term, "broadcasting," and gave us the world of instantaneous mass communication.[27] Moreover, technical and engineering factors alone, operating on the supply side of the equation, seldom dictate the ultimate "output" of new technology. Rather, this is something determined as much by consumer preference, demand expressed and orchestrated through markets. It is more useful to view basic science and technological innovation not as directly coupled, but as sharing similar but separate upward trajectories that are "interactive but semiautonomous."[28] Each influences the other in unpredictable ways. The notion of "use-inspired research" most often links science and technology with the promise of new processes and products, which experience, since the nineteenth century, has fixed in the public mind as realizable. In no field has it fixed itself more tenaciously than in medicine and health care. Within its subset, clinical and translational science expresses the urgency more keenly yet of squaring judgments about research promise with social need and urges better understanding of the role of use-inspired science.[29]

At the broadest institutional level, this was the significance of the NIH itself in the decades following World War II, its growth driven by three related factors. One was the public appetite for more and better medicine, an appetite that in time transformed medicine as understood as a vocation and service into health care recognized as an entitlement. Second was the presence of a highly self-confident medical profession that held its principles, if not always its practice, to be thoroughly "scientific." Third was the faith, shared by public and professionals alike, that use-inspired basic research moved everyone closer to the goal of less sickness and better health.[30] That basic science serves societal needs and desires appears a straightforward enough idea. When set against the reality of how science can be the source of desirable, but unpredictable, technological breakthroughs, its interactive nature becomes clear as well.[31]

Sometimes science and scientists proceed with no practical purpose in mind other than the solving of intellectual puzzles—something that fairly well describes James Watson and Francis Crick's famous work in unraveling the structure of DNA. It was practical, use-inspired interests, however, that led to Oswald Avery's discovery that DNA carried the genetic code. Subsequently, no field more than molecular biology demonstrates the interactive, multipath, mutually reinforcing relationships between science and technology. The use-inspired research at the heart of translation rests on this fact. In fields of science that bear on societal needs—and none does more so more urgently than medicine—the boundary between basic and use-inspired research blurs completely and rightly so. Given the indeterminate nature of scientific and technological development in the future, any basic research may possibly serve useful ends and may possibly not. Research that is not random but informed from the outset by the potential for use improves the odds that it will in fact do so and makes capturing the benefits in technology more likely.[32]

Commerce and Science

Translating science into medicine specifically and doing it more quickly and with better targeting is one chapter in the history of the commercialization of scientific ideas that covers many fields, including most famously in the modern era, chemistry, aircraft, and computers. In medicine, it is a story heavily weighted toward the recent end of the timeline.[33] For a century, taking ideas and discoveries of science to the clinic referred largely to pharmaceuticals, x-ray technology, and a few mechanical devices. Drug therapy dates to antiquity, although *de novo* synthesis waited on key advances in chemistry in the second half of the nineteenth century. The first synthetic pre-packaged drug was marketed in 1883. Penicillin was discovered in 1928 and put to stunning clinical use in the 1940s. Cimetidine, developed in the 1950s, revolutionized treatment for gastric and duodenal ulcer and went on to become the first "blockbuster" drug with $1 billion annual sales worldwide.[34] The biotechnology industry, which dates only from the 1970s with the founding of Genentech to develop biotherapeutics, represented a milestone event in the story of science and technological innovation, marking as it did not just the further application of science to industrial processes but also the essential convergence of science and business itself.[35]

Research and Development Expenditures
by Health-Care Sector, Percent of Revenues

SECTOR	SECTOR REVENUES	R AND D AS % OF REVENUES
Pharmaceutical	$200 billion	12–14%
Biotech	75 billion	15–20%
Medical Technology	140 billion	10–20%
Services (hospitals, clinics, extended care facilities, physicians)	1.6 trillion	Almost nothing

Source: Health Care Investment Group, *The Economist*, 2012; Statista.com.

Business cannot trade what it cannot value, which requires turning the ideas of science into forms of property. Patents accomplish this. In response to anxiety over declining global competitiveness of American industry, changes occurred in patent law beginning with the Bayh-Dole Act of 1980, which for the first time permitted universities to retain ownership of intellectual property developed with federal funding. Previously, ownership of discoveries made with federal support had belonged to the government, cutting off industry from a rich source of innovation and leaving inventors with low-to-zero incentive to seek to commercialize and profit from their work. Few did. Since Bayh-Dole, however, academic research institutions and their faculty turned the protection and development of intellectual property into significant lines of business, as universities found themselves in the business of business as they had never been before. Full-bore intrusion of business values into academe was a bracing and confusing experience. Some reveled in it; others recoiled.

Under the new incentives to protect and commercialize intellectual property, university patent filings soared. A new phrase—"technology transfer"—entered the academic vocabulary, and Offices of Technology Transfer became as ubiquitous as the offices of academic deans and provosts. Sometimes, this resulted in cooperation with existing companies (as has thus far been the case with funding for most translational research). More often, it turned out to lead to the formation of new business firms. Since 1980, more than 5,000 new businesses have sprung up as university-originated innovation moved out of laboratory into the reach of the marketplace and consumers.[36]

Not all innovative ideas are created equal, and different technologies, if they are to "transfer" into the world of commerce, face different opportunities and encounter different levels of risk along the way. Software and computing demands, for instance, differ significantly from biomedical therapeutics. With software, risk is back-loaded, meaning that while the technical risk is low, development times short, and intellectual property protected through copyright, instances still abound in which new products were launched but failed to find life in the market. On the other hand, risk is front-loaded with patent-protected therapeutics that must surmount arduous FDA barriers, making them harder to bring to market by a significant order of magnitude. Medical devices also face the barrier of entry of clinical proof and uncertain market adoption (although because they are more engineering than biology based, the development-stage barriers are less formidable). Diagnostics are at least as difficult to commercialize as therapeutics, requiring similarly extensive and expensive clinical testing but with generally narrower market opportunities. In all technology transfer, it is this ratio—between the cost of development and the potential revenue streams—that determines the chances of attracting investment and achieving successful commercialization.[37]

Academe, however intellectually open and committed to publication and knowledge-sharing, is a limited sphere. Industry, although proprietary and closed in the sense that it must be protective of shareholders' interests, is as broad as the market allows, and the broader the better. The collaboration that drives the commercialization of health care innovations depends on satisfying the different but complementary needs of academe and industry and deploying their different but complementary capabilities. Historically, academic science moves at its own internally determined rate. The financial, management, and marketing assets of industry can potentially accelerate it and, doing so, advance academic health centers' traditional three-pronged mission of research, education, and patient care (and more recently community service). To the benefit of industry, it has been argued that collaboration with AHCs offers access to a living laboratory unlike anything available in the business world alone.[38] AHCs already encompass (individually in miniature, collectively at some scale) the two most important stakeholders in the larger health care economy: patients and providers, in the form of physicians, nurses, and other clinical professionals. AHCs possess and, when working well, daily elaborate upon expertise across many fields and, when their various activities are added-up, broad clinical context. Industry requires a controllable setting for planning, testing, and validation of hoped-for commercial products, and AHCs can provide that setting. Levels of engagement between industry and AHCs range from simple consulting agreements, through sponsored research support (funding support often in return for licensing options), to forthright licensing transactions whereby an outside firm pays a fee for the right to commercialize an AHC's intellectual property, to larger scale strategic alliances.[39]

Liberated by Bayh-Dole, academic health-care entrepreneurs have learned how to navigate a path to commercialization that would be familiar to generations of entrepreneurs who came before them. They must be able to describe, beyond the intellectual/scientific merits of an idea, the market need and the real-world problem that their invention solves and then frame it as a value proposition. The technology itself must be understood in terms of its potential scope: Is it a platform technology or something in the category of an incremental improvement? The costs of development will then vary accordingly. Following on the research, health-care entrepreneurs must then ask is there a convincing pathway to development? The property must be protected against imitators: No one would invest in something that they cannot own.[40] Venture investors particularly see themselves in the primary business of assessing risk that they offset by setting high thresholds for return on their investment. Such targets cannot be met without a business plan built on sustained competitive market share and high margins and delivered by management versed in both science and the business of science. To commercialization prospects that involve human subjects must be added additional calculations around the relationship between innovation and safety. Finally, conflicts of interest and matters of divided loyalties must also be codified and managed.[41]

The Research/Enterprise Zone: New Middle Ground

On the best of days, effective translation confronts daunting institutional limitations and legacies. "We can no longer continue to operate the way we did in years past, with the model of one scientist in his or her lab doing his or her own thing."[42] So the director of what is probably the leading drug discovery program at a major research university worries that AHCs still, fundamentally, approach and practice basic science as they did fifty years ago and more. And this is so at the very moment when, at the other end of the translation pipeline, industry and pharmaceutical companies most need the unique science capability that AHCs represent but too frequently fail to convey.

Pharmacologist Jeff Conn's own elliptical career illustrates. After graduate school, he followed a conventional academic path and worked first in a NIH-driven university laboratory setting in a conservative medical center averse to the levels of investment and risk requisite to the success of larger endeavors. The better venue, he thought, for taking cutting-edge science and translating it into therapeutics was industry, and at Merck where he would eventually become head of neuroscience at the company's West Point, Pennsylvania, research facility near Philadelphia. Conn engaged in discovery work on new drugs for schizophrenia, Parkinson's disease, and chronic pain. Exciting as it was to be able to take programs to the point of clinical development and be able to answer questions of efficacy, the industry held its own frustrations. Some of the most exciting opportunities tend to be high risk, and companies shy away from the basic research needed to prove them out. This is precisely the kind of basic research at which universities excel.

Traditionally, there are two ways to work in discovery: either in academics where one does basic research but likely never really moves things forward, or in industry where different incentives often relegate promising fields to the sidelines for want of data. Neither situation suits optimum translation. In academe, there are cultural barriers to the way science is done that don't fit in with drug discovery, including funding and barriers related to how academics are promoted and rewarded and how they measure their own self-worth. The disparity is especially glaring between the historic individualist ethos of the academic laboratory and the large team efforts that are required for drug discovery in the twenty-first century. Conn probably understates that most university-based biomedical investigators do not understand truly large-scale collaborative science for the simple reason that most have never engaged in it. Many may have "collaborated"—with a colleague in a different department and shared authorship of a subsequent journal publication. Relatively few, however, have experienced research in large teams composed of multiple world-class experts where no individual succeeds outside reference to the team's effort. The distance between this and the by-now classical template of the NIH-funded principal investigator directing the efforts of post-docs and graduate students is hard to exaggerate. "You hear NIH talking a lot about large multidisciplinary collaborative science," Conn observes. "And you hear institutions talking about it. But when it comes right down to it, they don't fully understand or grasp it."[43]

The shortfall grows more critical as science improves. The process of drug discovery itself—finding drug targets, identifying lead compounds, testing in a preclinical environment and clinical studies, obtaining FDA approval, and then *perhaps* achieving successful entry into the marketplace—has remained remarkably constant over the years. It grows more complex, however. Genomics, proteomics, genetic association, and reverse genetics increase the ability to identify potential targets. High-throughput screening and combinatorial chemistry enhance the lead identification process. Better prediction of human drug pharmacokinetics due to advances in informatics and biotechnology improves lead optimization. The stages of clinical testing, while highly regulated with development requirements specifically defined by FDA code, meanwhile must accommodate the challenges of advancing discovery, as small-molecule agents with known pharmacologic mechanisms are joined by more novel structures derived from biotechnology.[44] The FDA's "critical path initiative," laid out in 2004 and modified two years later, aims at applying better tools (enhanced biomarker development, streamlined clinical trials, greater use of simulation and modeling) to improving actual product development and thus increasing the rate of flow in the drug discovery pipeline.[45] As they accumulate, such advances more and more demand the attention of teams of talent.

This is difficult for universities and is not perfectly executed in industry either. Conn describes what AHCs at their best can do to drive translation. "We're developing molecules that have all the properties that would make them viable as compounds that *could* be developed into drugs, and we're using those then to go into animal models and show that this is a viable approach. Then we publish that." The interest among academic scientists in pushing toward therapeutics must be present, but it is not sufficient. There must be outside partners who are prepared to invest and go the distance. In one example, Conn reports the instance of early discovery type work for a drug study that by its nature did not fit well into NIH study sections. A private company interested in this particular target and willing to fund the research then stepped in and, because it could not afford to develop internally the necessary research capability, proposed collaboration. The resulting university-generated, company-funded data was shared with no other strings attached. The company obtained results but, perhaps more important, they collected a great deal of data. In another instance, focused more sharply on drug discovery that would have breakthrough effects in patients, the university still maintained the freedom to publish. Yet where the goal is an actual drug—*technology transferred* to the market, no longer just the process of *technology transfer*—the intellectual property must be protected early, and scholars must be careful never to publish or otherwise disclose prematurely.

Industry needs information to make investment decisions, and AHCs can but do not always supply it. Conn recounts, how when working in industry, he saw all kinds of interesting ideas coming from academic institutions, but most were "kind of half-baked." While a proposal might look potentially innovative and high impact, there was typically seldom enough data to enable a solid conclusion as to its viability much less enough data to convince top corporate leadership. Too often, for example, an academic scientist may identify a gene expressed in a cancer cell with a receptor that could be a drug target. He writes a paper suggesting that this would be a good drug target for this particular cancer. The head of a cancer department in a large drug company might look at the paper and think it interesting, but then groan at the amount of effort required to investigate. To do so might require dedicating a significant portion of his department to the task—one which would be highly speculative with high risk of failure. "And there are hundreds of such speculative ideas out there every day," says Conn.[46]

At a large pharmaceutical company, nothing is deemed successful unless it goes all the way to market. If it does not go the entire distance—a very big "if"—it is "at the end of the day a failure."[47] There are instances where drugs pass through phase two proof of concept and, in some cases, even phase three and have established efficacy, yet are still abandoned because predicted market penetration is not high enough to justify full development and roll-out. Moreover, what happens after "failure" can compound the loss, as an entire field of investigation may be abandoned. Reviving a failed program in a large pharmaceutical company is all but impossible, even if it is a program where much has been learned and there is a probability of success in a subsequent investigation. Worse—for science and the prospect of translation—is the risk-averse instinct then to lock away the findings against the possibility that someone else might happen on the "something that is there but that we just don't know about yet" and pursue it successfully.[48]

On the middle ground of a Research/Enterprise Zone, the bar would be set differently. Success can, for instance, mean proving a negative. If researchers publish the results of good science that shows this or that approach will never work for therapeutic agents, then that is a lauded in academe and contributes to the world of science generally. Such "failure" is also a success for the greater translational endeavor and for industry, which must do most of the heavy lifting as discovery approaches its ultimate goal, where a substance can be tested and perhaps proved effective in humans. Such knowledge may save half a dozen companies enormous time, energy, and money otherwise wasted down blind alleys and dead ends. Once corporate/scientific decisionmakers knows where *not* to look and are enabled by the levels of data that confirm truly viable approaches, "then they have something to go with. They know exactly how to go about making those molecules, because you've paved the way."[49]

What is needed is protected and incentivized team science, advanced enough to supply the data that industry demands and can depend on, *and* that is prepared to take up challenges that industry discards. It is a rare and delicate ecology. AHCs of a certain temperament, or spaces set off and protected within them, would be the best candidates to take up this role, one that would operate in between traditional academic and traditional industry research. Traditional academe is filled with too many lone wolves, whether plodders or stars, and a reward system centered on tenure and the prestige of publication—rather than the prospect of wealth with the promise of permanence. The traditional industry represented by large pharma operates under business constraints that make it hard to risk the financial resources that promising, problem-based basic research requires, and a reward system widely criticized as skewed to the short term. Given competition and normal market incentives however, business innovates naturally or dies. Firms that forget the lessons of past experience fail to adapt and grow old before their time. New, nimble ones emerge. To such prods academe is largely a stranger.

Twenty-first century AHCs exist partly within academe and partly outside it and are candidates at least to occupy this middle space. To do so, they must establish and sustain conditions friendly to team-driven translational research that is tailored specifically to industry needs. A culture of faculty and administrative collegiality already operates in many places and is a product of intangible forces that cannot be mandated. To encourage such an environment, there must be funding enough to recruit and retain intellectual capital, and not just top talent from elsewhere in academe but from industry, from among people who already know how to do great discovery. There must be funding to acquire and renew the capital-intensive physical infrastructure of major core facilities. And at top leadership levels, there must be entrepreneurial expertise and energy of a caliber at least matching that found in the most innovative private industries. It will be challenging ground for legacy institutions to capture and harder yet to hold.

Or, it may be time for a new model entirely that could manage more directly the fundamental clash between business and academic cultures, cultures with their own values, rules, and priorities. It is difficult for academic institutions to grapple with this issue and such reluctance can cripple progress toward speeding the conversion of knowledge into service. The clash surrounds compensation, secrecy and publishing, the protection of intellectual property, and the rights of the academic commons. A new organizational entity might be preferable, possibly beginning with joint ventures within university settings but insulated in ways that would secure different rules of engagement with the goal of maximizing successful collaboration with industry.

Business Barriers

It is a fine feeling to be of use—what Abraham Flexner said he most wanted in life and the legacy to which he aspired.[50] In contemporary language, the equivalent phrase is "making a difference," and it is the reason that young people universally give for seeking out medical education and the reason that validates the career choice of medical practitioners everywhere. However, science makes a difference in medicine only if translated. Viewed as the foundation of translation, science can be hard for universities because it sometimes seems too applied. It can be equally hard for business. Translational research narrowly defined can be too distant, too far from commercialization and the clinical impact to attract needed capital. Biomedical science in general presents obstacles for business that have retarded performance of the biotech and pharmaceutical industries and have yet to be convincingly and consistently overcome. Until they are, being "of use" will not mean what it one day might. Three characteristics of science challenge business as it attempts to take up translation.[51]

First, the uncertainty and therefore the risk are greater. All research and development entails the risk of unknown outcomes, but biomedical research and development must contend with primary uncertainty, the problem not of known but of unknown unknowns.[52] Will a desired experimental result yield something that is even remotely feasible technically? The movie business is an example of research and development done on a daily basis. Most firms fail, but with those few that don't there is no question about how it is they will "work." This is different, for instance, from research and development aimed at finding cures for cancer, where scientific "breakthroughs" do not necessarily translate easily or soon to commercial applications of early use to patients. They may just as likely point to the need for more rounds of yet newer research down heretofore un-guessed-at paths, and time horizons are always long. The work is slow and unpredictable. Even the work done thus far to unravel the human genome, touted by the media as a "revolution," remains in the earliest stages, more on the taxiway than the runway to clinical utility.

All businesses, if they are to stay in business, must learn to manage the risks of uncertainty. But the sort of primary risks attending the business of biomedicine and biotechnology raise the stakes. The business mechanisms that in modern economies have evolved to manage and measure risk—from private and public equity markets and venture capital to contractual and institutional arrangements like licensing and patents—in essence convert the intangibles of ideas, innovations, and know-how into intellectual property that can be monetized and thus moved about. This process can however er create barriers to the knowledge-sharing at the heart of good science. Ultimately, one hopes that more and better knowledge, which is what research produces, will reduce uncertainty and therefore lower business risk.[53]

Second, it is a truism that science is complex. The changes of the last thirty years have seen this complexity compounded in a way that additionally challenges the uptake of science by business. If this has been a time of "revolutions" (molecular, genomic, proteomic), they have been multiple and diverse and are as interrelated and as oddly formed as the closely fitting pieces of a jigsaw puzzle. The kinds of understanding needed even to begin to discern the picture they have revealed has broadened apace. Until the 1970s, classical drug discovery as pursued by large pharmaceutical firms, and in the university laboratories that fed them, relied largely on medicinal chemistry. Today, drug discovery demands competence across new disciplines that are themselves works in progress: bioinformatics, combinatorial chemistry, cell biology, and others. Successful development of new therapeutics depends more than ever on sharing and integrating knowledge across diverse endeavors and organizational boundaries—a huge learning opportunity but an equal challenge to business. The need to share and integrate information is hardly unique to the business of drug discovery, but whereas some complex products can be thought of as composed of discrete modular parts (a computer or an airliner, for instance), this is not yet so in the biological sciences. The way information and experts in diverse biomedical fields come together is still largely *ad hoc* and a long way from anything resembling a system.[54] Moreover, very little biomedical knowledge is easily reduced to precise meanings and widely applicable principles, at least not at first glance. In the work of drug discovery, much knowledge remains tacit in nature (not easily described by those who possess it), embedded in experience and judgment, even instinct. Teams of researchers best share collective experience, although the tendency, as seen in academic laboratories or in the proliferation of new firms in the biotechnology industry, is to form "specialized expertise islands" that impede knowledge integration.[55]

Third, because biomedical science is so turbulent and the risks to successful commercialization so great, the need for active, never-ending learning is paramount for all involved. "Dancing on the edge of knowledge," as the activity of the drug-discovery industry has been described, makes for many decisions that may be best at the moment but inevitably prove not to be the right ones, or only partially the right ones. Failures outnumber successes, always. Organizations learn from their mistakes in different ways and at different levels, sometimes individually and haphazardly, other times organizationally and more formally. Different organizations, even those making the same thing, like General Motors and Toyota, learn differently and with wide variations of the effectiveness of their memories on the quality of their products and ultimately on the value of their business.[56] Until biomedicine and biotechnology firms learn to improve the institutionalization of learning, much will (continue to) be lost or, at best, mislaid. This will not be easy and indeed may conflict with other concurrent business needs, such as the need to manage risk.

University Possibilities

When Abraham Flexner stipulated in 1910 that a chief condition for the reform of medical education (and the funding of that reform) was that medical schools henceforth be joined organically to universities, he had both substantive and reputational issues in mind. Up to then, the training of physicians, as the practice of medicine itself, often as not operated as small businesses typically undercapitalized and poorly managed. The pervasively low scientific standards of many such school and businesses meant that they produced a broad stream of equally substandard practitioners who further depressed the reputation of the profession. Science even at that point was capable of much better, as a handful of university-based schools already had demonstrated, if such methods could be effectively brought to bear on medical education. To anchor medical education within the realm of the university, as Flexner prescribed, was to expunge once and for all the stain of bad, old proprietary days: insurance against intellectual mediocrity and guaranteeing the central place of science. (Anchors assure stability by retarding movement. Depending on the need at the moment, this can be either desirable or, literally, a drag. To restore forward movement, it may be necessary to up anchor; see chapter six). That done, the scientifically-educated doctors produced at reformed university-based medical schools became beneficiaries twice over of the scientific research that also was to occur there. From the presence of researchers practicing in their midst, these doctors of the 1920s, 1930s, and 1940s absorbed a reverence for practical bench research as an important key to helping patients. It was also assumed that such university-trained medical men (and a few women) would become the natural carriers, into practice, of the insights that science had brought to medicine—that they would become the translators of medicine as science into medicine as service. This proved true enough, if only for the time when the delivery of care was relatively simple, in terms of low demand and low cost.

The universities into which Flexner said medical schools must be embedded still at that time dwarfed their new medical appendages, in a relationship of power and influence he had no way of foreseeing would someday be turned on its head. In fact, both higher education and university medical centers (which became academic health centers) were destined to become big businesses each on their own, though not-for-profit ones. And both were destined to follow down the paths where their researchers led and to become involved in earnest in the business of science.

The dimension of this return to the marketplace might have perplexed Flexner. In 2003, Harvard Medical School and Massachusetts General Hospital had licensing revenues of $46 million (half from one biotech drug, Enbrel). Columbia University earned upwards of $300 million over twenty years from the "Axel" patents on recombinant DNA technology.[57] It became not uncommon for many universities to take on roles as active venture investors, assuming equity stakes, and risks, in faculty-originated start-ups. In some cases, it was early-stage activity in biomedical research, but sometimes universities ventured downstream as well, into commercial drug development and testing. All these ventures added up. In 2007, American academic research institutions reported signing more than 5,000 licenses and options and the startup of more than 500 new companies. More than 3,000 past startups were still in business, and licensees had brought close to 700 new products to market. Each headline—"Tuberculosis Vaccine May Save Millions of Lives" (Albert Einstein College of Medicine); "Silver-based Pharmaceutical Candidates to Treat Infections and Cancer" (University of Akron); "Building a Surgical Device Business" (University of Arkansas for Medical Sciences); "LabNow Revolutionizes HIV/AIDS Treatment" (University of Texas at Austin)[58]—told a unique story but with common roots in the altruism and the ambition of inventors and institutions. And each produced, in its own unique mixture, the private gain and public benefit that lie at the heart of capitalism.

It has been argued that heavy emphasis in universities on maximizing returns from licensing revenue and equity investing, much in the same spirit as the monetization of intellectual property in the biotechnology business, erodes the scientific commons that remains critical to further fundamental advance in biomedicine and the translation of research into the development of useful therapeutics.[59] The high, some would say hyper, sensitivity about conflicts of interest that today attends the mixing of academic and business endeavors attests to profound insecurity on this issue. One can imagine Flexner raising such cautions. One can also imagine him probing hard for the proper relationship between universities and industry in the field of biomedicine, certain that the relationship must evolve and certain that the service of medicine, as reinvigorated by science in the twentieth century, must in the twenty-first century be spread by all means at hand including perhaps even especially by business. Perhaps, the time has come for less anchor and more sail.

Terms and Conditions

A century after Flexner's report, health care had become an enormous public/private edifice housing a tangle of science and service. Some saw this as a shameful bedlam, others as a proud feat. No one, least of all Flexner, would not agree that it was proof at least of needs unmet—for more knowledge, fresh structures, ever-better leadership. Mindful of the complexity of technology commercialization in university settings, there is good evidence of the conditions that can smooth the junction between academe and industry and shape the most effective transfer processes. These are the same requirements that, in all technology, transfer and feed economic development, and that in health care can heighten the impact of science on the service of medicine. Clearly, not everything works everywhere. Academic institutions famously guard their individuality, often to excess. Entrepreneurs are nothing if not individuals, often fiercely so. But we have learned enough to understand that what sparks transfer everywhere, and sustains it past the first hand-offs, is science, support, leadership, and culture in strong and equal measure.

Often what sounds obvious is most easily missed. The most effective transfer depends on the most effective science, qualitatively of course but also quantitatively. Research abhors isolation and thrives on company. Magnitude matters: Broad and brimming pipelines are best. The most successful universities build strong research bases deliberately and do not rely on the assumed additive effects of the interests of individual scientists alone. They plan research strategically around core-, already-realized or potentially-realizable in the near term, institutional competencies. To be most effective, such strategies must also seek to align competencies (supply) with emerging trends in the market for particular kinds of products and service (demand). This done, they recruit top, "star" talent to be magnets for others and for further funding. Federal research and development funding is targeted, and centers of excellence developed and promoted intramurally and made visible outside campus walls. Top ranking in NIH funding is a benchmark of leadership in successful transfer for medical research institutions. Rankings are closely watched, and winning the improvement of a notch or two up the ladder is the aim of every dean and vice president for medical affairs. Membership in the elite "top ten" is the best club of all.

NIH Top Ten Research Institutions, 2014

INSTITUTION	RANK	RESEARCH FUNDING
University of California San Francisco	1	$441,676,083
Johns Hopkins University	2	$404,918,256
University of Pennsylvania	3	$379,380,010
Stanford University	4	$314,801,445
Yale University	5	$311,824,870
Washington University	6	$298,483,750
University of Pittsburgh	7	$297,016,461
University of Washington	8	$293,161,597
Vanderbilt University	9	$292,413,440
Duke University	10	$284,982,977

Source: Blue Ridge Institute for Medical Research, 2014.

Adjacency of leadership in other fields and schools can also be critical. Consider three examples.[60] Stanford regularly ranks among top ten medical schools. Its graduate school of business regularly ranks even higher (number one or two, typically), and its school of engineering enrolls a quarter of all Stanford students, a share second only to MIT. Graduate programs in biology and chemistry rank near the nation's top. Seventeen Stanford faculties boast Nobels and 133 are member of the National Academy of Sciences.[61] In 1970, Stanford pioneered establishment of an office of technology licensing, which actively marketed its protected intellectual property to promising licensees. The patenting of recombinant DNA, with its handsome financial returns, was just the most famous example of the success of its approach. Stanford also holds equity positions in numerous faculty-originated start-ups, which in order to mitigate potential conflict it sells as soon as allowed and well before they approach top return.[62] After Frederick Terman's "steeples of excellence" policy on faculty hiring from the 1960s, the university consistently sought out the best talent on the market but with the stipulation that it support its own research activities. In medicine, this meant NIH funding but not that alone, and research conducted with supplemental or even primary industry support was encouraged and rewarded. More and more and younger and younger faculty could be found taking leaves of absence in order to work in industry, mostly in start-ups or young firms. Stanford's president himself once took leave to start a company. A relentless back-and-forth between business and university is common at all levels, as is part-time consulting to industry.

Development of an entrepreneurial culture was not however left to individual faculty initiative alone. Formal teaching of entrepreneurship, supported by corporations and venture capitalists and drawing on alumni and the community for faculty resources (read Silicon Valley) suffused the curriculum with courses, work-studies, and practical internships. The Stanford Technologies Ventures Programs centered in the engineering school enrolled primarily not only business students but also prospective engineers and scientists. The Business Association for Stanford Engineering Students (BASES), with 5,000 members half from current students and faculty and half from business executives, venture capitalists, and others in the business community, became the largest entrepreneurship organization in the country. In addition to practical programs on start-ups and business plan development, BASES promoted student-run business plan competitions. The Entrepreneur's Challenge competition has categories in hardware, software, and biomedicine, and teams, not individuals, compete for a $25,000 grand prize. A yearly Innovation Showcase hosted jointly with the University of California, Berkeley, attracts industry and venture capital audiences. Networking is endemic and hardwired through interschool and department technology panels, opportunities to play "venture capitalist for a night," and local venture capitalists and attorneys who provide *pro bono* counseling to would-be entrepreneurs. Reaching back to the 1950s, Terman had promoted the continuing education at Stanford of working engineers drawn to the then-young transistor and semiconductor industries. It is notable that no one agency coordinates these activities, although the activities themselves are deliberate, highly intentional, and in that sense strategic on the part of the university. Innovation and discovery are things worked at though never exactly planned. In the Stanford instance, an abundance of (largely federal) research funding, plus sustained intramural effort to validate and reward the pursuit of commercial opportunity, plus the ready presence of private investment capital, business infrastructure, and know-how, has bred enviable rates of innovation and technology transfer. It might be called a strategic culture of entrepreneurship.

The University of Pennsylvania, with research and development expenditures more than $700 million (2003), 80 percent federally funded and 70 percent dealing with life sciences, accomplishes comparable performance but over a somewhat different path.[63] Also a top-ten research university, Penn boasts a top-ten medical school as well as the renowned Wharton School of Business, plus twenty-five research centers and institutes including the interdisciplinary Institute for Medicine and Engineering, and the Management and Technology Program, an offshoot of the Wharton School and the school of engineering. Penn's Center for Technology Transfer (CTT) in 2003 ranked in the second quartile for new patents issued, licenses, and start-ups and in the first quartile for license income. Between 1996 and 2003, its technology transfer activities generated an average return on investment of just under 200 percent.

As it has evolved since 1986, CTT manages the chain of activities that lead from invention disclosure all the way to the start-up of actual firms. The center's staff first triages faculty disclosures and conducts due diligence. Wharton MBA students do market research. Management and Technology Program students from Wharton and the engineering school look at an invention's commercial potential. Using external consultants, CTT then works out business models and hires professional management. It is the newly hired CEO who then secures financing. Penn faculty and staff may work as advisors and consultants but may not exercise management or fiduciary roles. Thirty percent of the income received from commercialization returns to the inventor, with the same amount split evenly between the inventor's laboratory and home academic department. (The rest goes to the inventor's school, the university's research foundation and a small intellectual property fund.) CTT sometimes facilitates what it does not directly manage, as in the role it played in helping to establish a cooperative drug-discovery partnership between Penn's school of medicine and the pharmaceutical firm GlaxoSmithKline. It also supports a Translational Research Facility of 120,000 square feet of life science laboratories adjacent to its own offices and plans a multi-acre research park nearby. Working closely with the university, the Commonwealth of Pennsylvania supports complementary structures in support of entrepreneurial development and technology transfer, and with $100 million of tobacco settlement funds established three Life Sciences Greenhouses. One of them, "BioAdvance," specializes in early stage and proof of concept projects in biotherapeutics, diagnostics, devices, and tools, and judge proposals on three areas: commercial opportunity, technical merit, and intellectual property. Three additional state-originated funds, PA Early

Stage Partners, Quaker BioVentures, and Birchmere Ventures, each requiring 3:1 private/public matching, created a $180 million pool of seed capital.

State initiatives can be as fickle as the legislatures that pass them, but when sustained they can help create an environment that makes university establishment of space for technology transfer easier. At Penn, it was critical that highest-level executive leadership make the case for the linkage of technology transfer to local and regional economic development. This required new structures inside the university (at Penn, the Office of Strategic Initiatives) and active promotion of the linkage to stakeholders in every school and department of the university and to constituents in the outside community. With its diversity of universities, other research organizations and corporations, the Philadelphia example demonstrated the multiplier opportunity for technology alliances where so much of the work of research and commercialization (and certainly all of it in biomedicine) required integration across multidisciplinary fields.

It can take bold and steadfast university leadership to promote commercialization over ingrained institutional suspicion about the compatibility of academic life and technology transfer (and the rewards attendant to it). At least one historical example illustrates how, if commercialization is rooted firmly enough in the ethos and language of service to society, suspicion dissipates quickly, and the technology transfer enterprise moves from the margin to the center of an institution's mission.

The University of Wisconsin boasts the country's oldest technology transfer program, founded in 1925 squarely on the principle that research enables medicine as service.[64] The Wisconsin Alumni Research Foundation (WARF) began in order to manage faculty biochemist Harry Steenbock's work with vitamin D, which led to elimination of the disease rickets. As a federal land grant institution, the University of Wisconsin's heritage of concern for social welfare and economic development went back even farther than that and exemplified the commitment of teaching, research and service to communities across the state made famous by Senator Robert La Follette and known to history as "The Wisconsin Idea."

WARF functions as an independent but university-linked nonprofit technology and development organization. It files patents, issues licenses, and promotes commercialization of inventors' innovations, and it is liberal with ownership rights and rewards. Except where federal funding is involved, inventors receive 20 percent of royalties, the inventor's laboratory 70 percent. WARF contributes large sums back to the university to support further research and development through grants and new facilities, including dedicated funds for the hiring of interdisciplinary faculty, its "cluster hire initiative." As in Pennsylvania, congenial state support complements WARF's backing for early-stage firms, investment vehicles for entrepreneurs, and funds university research infrastructure. Most licenses, in fact, go to companies outside Wisconsin, and WARF at one time kept a representative in San Diego charged with developing licensing and investing leads on the West Coast. While it was politically attractive and advantageous for some entrepreneurs to seek opportunities in the home state, the market ultimately governed. "You have to view the corporation as the customer," explained WARF's executive director in 2003, "We are selling [technology] to them; you've got to have high quality research but you also have to be talking to industry and have a presence."[65] In the early 1970s, WARF pushed the development limits too far and for a time lost its nonprofit status (later restored when it sold off its development laboratories). It continues however with an aggressive approach to licensing, patenting, and start-up activities.

Fully within the university, an Office of Corporate Relations (OCR) promotes contacts and a central point of entry with the corporate sector and focuses on matching university researchers to the requirements of specific business and corporate projects. A searchable database gives corporations detailed access to the university's research capabilities and services. Entrepreneurship education and development occurs through WARF, OCR, and Wisconsin's business school, where a Technology Innovation Fund (funded from licensing revenues from prior inventions) awards grants for proof of concept projects with patent and licensing potential. An Industrial and Economic Development Research Program provides additional support for early-stage research. In 1984, the university initiated a 300-acre research park with 1.5 million square feet, University Research Park, Inc., a self-sustaining nonprofit entity (no city or state subsidy, though property taxes are paid to the city). By the early 2000s, this research park hosted more than 100 new firms concentrated in biotechnology (with 4,000 employees and average salaries of $60,000), two-thirds of them with some connection to the university.

All factors combined—beginning with a strong research base particularly in the school of medicine, the aggressive WARF technology strategy of seeking out corporations as customers for university-generated research, liberality in rewarding inventors and the presence of an incubator-rich research park— increased the number of start-ups and promoted a cross-institutional enterprise culture.

Science, applied and valued through the marketplace, feels natural at Wisconsin, not exceptional. But as with examples of successful technology transfer elsewhere,[66] it depends on sustaining the right business and institutional culture. There must be a strong and strategically focused research base within the university to feed the process. University culture itself must reward not inhibit inventiveness and entrepreneurial behavior aimed at solving practical problems outside the walls. Technology transfer offices, by whatever name, must be active in forging relationships and in bringing together supply and demand—the key academic researchers and "customers" for their ideas in business and industry. They should foster management capabilities (or supply professional management) on the understanding that great researchers and great businessmen seldom occupy the same skin. They should have ties to sources of angel, philanthropic, and venture capital, and to potential industry collaborators who need guidance in how university research operates and where the best opportunities are to be found. First and last, champions—typically the executive leadership of universities and academic medical centers, with business as well as academic background—are needed to prod naturally sluggish institutions into new modes of action and to educate them in new possibilities for service through applied knowledge.[67]

To contribute, through technology, to the social good and to the economic welfare of the state and society may in Wisconsin be seen as a form of altruism and civic duty, the beneficent legacy of a unique history. In fact, it is the natural consequence of technology transfer properly understood and pursued, and of the business of science everywhere.

TWO

Making Truth Useful

D*iscovery* sounds new and exciting and always has. Just think of Christopher Columbus, so revered by Americans before the age of political correctness. Columbus "discovered America," we learned as schoolchildren, and so we celebrated every October 12 as his special day. Columbus was a brave risk-taker and innovator: He sailed west in order, he hoped, to reach the east and so demonstrated empirically that the world was round. Of greater immediate interest to Ferdinand and Isabella, his royal patrons, Columbus found a "new world" ripe for possession (no matter that he thought he was in China). And as his successors would soon confirm, it turned out to be a very rich new world indeed. Columbus was not of course the first European to find America, but he was the first one to make his finding known. The Vikings vanished into the northern mists: explorers but not discoverers. Columbus not only found America, but he returned to Europe with the news. That was when things started to happen.

It is like this in health care today. Biomedical research explores rich new worlds of understanding about how our bodies work (and how they don't), but we haven't acted effectively enough upon the news. So there is still a gap between our knowledge and our practice, between the best that discovery has made plain and the better health that still eludes us. Evidence-based medicine (EBM), the second component of a system of service, is the tool that helps us act upon discovery's knowledge and disciplines its day-to-day delivery.

Yet there is little within modern health care, at least within the health care professions themselves, that generates more contentious debate. All the old clichés prevail about whether medicine is primarily an art or a science.[1] At the extremes, evangelists see in EBM a momentous Thomas Kuhn-like "new paradigm" for health care: just do this and the world of medicine and health will be changed forever and greatly for the better. Skeptics warn darkly of positivist arrogance, lost professional (chiefly physician) autonomy, the triumph of "cookbook medicine," and the "McDonald's-ization" of a once-noble profession. We are wise to qualify these simplifying metaphors at the start.

The best cooks know that no recipe guarantees a great dish, and that cooking is akin to live performance in the arts where no two performances are ever exactly alike, though all may be equally superb. Great cooks keep a tasting spoon close at hand and make adjustments according to what tongue and nose tell them at the moment. So great doctors exercise clinical judgment, which is something they will have acquired in practice and that no protocol can teach. The pejorative "McDonald's-ization" also misses the mark. McDonald's delivers value much as it did when it first opened in the 1950s, with a low-priced menu designed to appeal to a broad market with simple tastes; fast service; brand power derived from remarkably consistent quality over thousands of worldwide locations. Process, not product, innovation has enabled the fast-food giant to do this and explains its business success. Medicine is obviously more complex than making burgers and fries, but much of it involves similarly repetitive processes. Just ask a family practitioner, or for that matter an orthopaedic surgeon who "does hips." In the real world, where medicine meets the market or navigates the entitlement regime, it is the process of delivery as much as the quality of the widely-agreed-upon recipes that becomes the critical issue. The claims surrounding EBM therefore need be neither utopian nor dystopian. "Mundane" will do.

Evidence-based medicine is the product of post–World War II intellectual and administrative developments in British and American medicine that elevated the randomized clinical trial as the standard by which therapeutic effectiveness could best be measured. It took root in Britain against the background of the launch of the National Health Service in the late 1940s, while the thalidomide scandal of the late 1950s and early 1960s, and the subsequent activism of the Food and Drug Administration in the United States and comparable agencies in other western countries gave it urgency. This occurred within the context of medicine's increasing centralization and bureaucratization generally, the changing (chiefly growing) role of government, and the pervasiveness of third-party payment, which ineluctably raised the pressure for uniformity and control of both doctors and hospitals.[2] And when it came (belatedly), concern over costs and the response of managed care regimes together made EBM a favored instrumentality for how diagnosis and standards of treatment would be evaluated and indeed enforced.

Evidence-based medicine—defined by one of its founders, epidemiologist David Sackett, as "the conscientious, explicit and judicious use of current best evidence in making decisions about the care of individual patients"—does in fact leads to better, more efficient care and broadly improved health outcomes.[3] It makes good physicians (and not physicians alone but all members of the health-care team) into better ones. It informs, but does not replace, clinical judgment. It strives both to streamline and regularize processes, and to vet the content of interventions that should or should not be applied in any given situation. It challenges unexamined reliance on professional judgment and idiosyncratic experience. It protects against medicine's old nemeses of theory and fads.

Evidence-based medicine is scientific management, figuratively at least, blended with clinical practice. It addresses deficits in scientific knowledge and attitudes that account for wildly variable practices and results across different populations and geographical areas, and it provides tools to measure the effectiveness and efficiency of interventions by giving practitioners quick access to the most current and highest-quality information in summary form. This is critical, because as biomedical discovery accelerates and translation improves, the individual medical professional's cognitive abilities diminish relatively. Summarizing, generalizing, and making usable best evidence—and then customizing it to the individual patient—is no longer just a preferred way to achieve and sustain improved outcomes. It is a possible and perhaps even a necessary one.

The root concept is hardly newer than inductive science itself. To observe and then to make something of the observation is the first step of science. Eighteenth- and nineteenth-century Paris was renowned for its great hospitals, which, while offering minimal therapy for patients, at least afforded clinicians of that day abundant opportunity systematically to observe sick people and from their observations seek out truths about their maladies. Some suggest that the roots of EBM, in the sense of somehow testing treatments for their efficacy, reach further back yet to eleventh-century Persia and Avicenna's *The Canon of Medicine*, to Aristotle's Athens, even to ancient China. For the beginnings of an evidence-based sensibility, nearer history points us to the movements for hospital standardization in the United States in the early twentieth century, to the coming of standardized paper-based patient records, to the standardization of medical education that followed Flexner's famous report, indeed to Frederick Taylor's quest for measurement and efficiency in American industry generally.

But whereas such earlier manifestations of the standardization idea tended to focus on tools, skills, and infrastructure, evidence-based guidelines and medicine, as it has emerged to prominence in the past thirty years, directly concerned itself with the *content* of what it is best to do. Whether or not this constitutes a "new paradigm," or is harbinger of "different worlds," as some have said, it certainly does constitute a radical intrusion into the way clinical medicine had traditionally been done in hospitals and doctors' offices everywhere.[4] That model, both before and after the therapeutic revolution of the 1940s and 1950s, had seen the individual doctor as the vessel of all knowledge and placed him (almost always "him" then) squarely at the center of things in every sense, as famously rendered graphically in the Luke Fildes 1891 painting *The Doctor*. It was a model where scientific knowledge sat on one side of the problem of the disease problem, the individual patient on the other. Only the trained, experienced doctor, exercising his hard-earned clinical judgment case by unique case, linked the two in each act of medical decision making. This made for medicine that was highly personalized in terms of the doctor-patient relationship and sometimes, but not always, scientific. It presumed paternalistic doctors and passive patients. Sometimes, it yielded good results, sometimes not.

Two developments have rendered this approach obsolete. Both were cumulative and both reached tipping points about the same time in the 1970s and 1980s. One was the quantum explosion of biomedical knowledge, much of it molecular in nature, which made earlier "breakthrough" periods in the history of medicine look modest by comparison. In order to deliver competent care, there was much more that it was necessary to know. The problem was that there was no more time for clinicians to know it. Second was the accumulation in daily practice of unacknowledged, often unrecognized bad work habits—the way in which too many doctors, while believing in the efficacy of science in medicine as much as anyone, nevertheless applied science to medicine day-to-day in ways that were frankly unscientific.

Evidence-based medicine, as the new approaches would be called, had multiple fathers. One was Englishman Archie Cochrane who first came upon signs of a problem in the use of certain medical interventions—used because they were available, not necessarily because they worked—while a medical officer among British soldiers in German POW camps during World War II. In one camp, where there was barely anything to work with, mortality rates were actually lower than in a second camp where facilities were notably better and where doctors had the wherewithal to offer better care. Was it possible, Cochrane wondered, that doing more while not knowing exactly what one was doing actually cost lives? He went on to evangelize for randomized, controlled clinical trials as the only reliable method to distinguish in the aggregate what was helpful from what was harmful. He also established the eponymous institute dedicated to the cause, the now-worldwide Cochrane Collaboration.[5] High-quality, quickly-accessible information based on such trials came to define the "evidence" that mattered most to medicine. Cochrane's American counterpart was epidemiologist John Wennberg. Since the 1990s, Wennburg's *Dartmouth Atlas of Health Care* has correlated the use of a variety of medical and surgical interventions with geographical occurrence to reveal, for instance, that the higher frequency of certain kinds of surgeries, which seemed medically inexplicable, occurred more frequently in a certain location due to greater availability of surgeons and diagnostics tests. Wennberg's famous maps illustrated the consequences of the inadequate use and sharing of the best-available knowledge—a systemic failure that gave wide leeway to idiosyncratic, sometimes unsafe and costly, physician practice styles. Cochrane and Wennberg were joined by Canadian and British epidemiologists David Sackett and Gordon Guyatt, who tackled methodological challenges of analyzing the vast quantities of data produced by clinical trials, to arrive at useable definitions of what constituted "best evidence"; Sackett and Guyatt are also usually credited with originating the term "evidence-based medicine" to describe the new approach.[6]

From then to now, the definition of EBM has remained faithful to its origins even while it has evolved. First formulations highlighted the care of *individual* patients.[7] Current ones add clinical expertise and patient values to the mix and expand the meaning of "evidence" beyond the so-called "gold standard" of randomized controlled trials to include other sorts of systematically acquired information.[8] David Eddy, the physician who wrote the first national guideline explicitly based on evidence and who was among the first to use the term "evidence-based," argues that the need for a unified approach of two distinct ideas is embedded in our understanding of EBM: evidence-based guidelines (EBG), which are generic and influence groups of providers (and not just doctors) and individual patients indirectly, and evidence-based individual decision making (EBIM), which focuses on individual physicians learning to apply evidence-based methods on individual patients.[9] For now, "Evidence-based practice as the integration of *best research evidence* with *clinical expertise* and *patient values*" expresses the consensus understanding where terms are carefully defined:

- "Best research evidence" refers to clinically relevant research, often from the basic health and medical sciences, but especially from patient-centered clinical research into the accuracy and precision of diagnostic tests (including the clinical examination); the power of prognostic markers; and the efficacy and safety of therapeutic, rehabilitative, and preventive regimens.

- "Clinical expertise" means the ability to use clinical skills and past experience to identify rapidly each patient's unique health state and diagnosis, individual risks and benefits of potential interventions, and personal values and expectations.

- "Patient values" refer to the unique preferences, concerns, and expectations that each patient brings to a clinical encounter and that clinicians must integrate into clinical decisions if they are to serve the patient."[10]

Given future refinements and the inevitable tinkering with terminology, what hasn't changed thus far and almost certainly won't is the primacy of "integration." Unless it all happens together, all of the time, no amount of evidence will change outcomes.

The graphic commonly used to depict integration is a Venn diagram; in this diagram of three interlocking circles, one represents the doctor's individual clinical experience; one the best external evidence; and one patient values and expectations. The relatively small area where the three overlap represents the area of "evidence-based medicine."[11] Compared to the larger circles themselves, it is a small but well-filled space. This is where evidence-based medicine happens according to a sequence of actions now widely taught in medical school. First, convert information needs into answerable questions. Then, track down the best evidence to answer these questions. Then, appraise that evidence for its validity and usefulness. Next, apply the results in practice. Finally, evaluate your own performance and improve next time.

The Evidence-based Medicine Triad

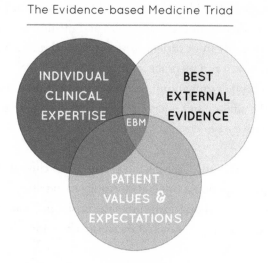

Source: Florida State University, College of Medicine;
http://med.fsu.edu/index.cfm?page=medicalinformatics.
ebmTutorial. Retrieved October 7, 2015.

It has been a dangerous temptation to evaluate the influence of clinical practice guidelines—"systematically developed statements to assist practitioner and patient decisions about appropriate health care for specific clinical circumstances"[12]—primarily against their adoption by individual health professionals, particularly doctors. On the one hand, proliferating thousands of guidelines can come to look like just so much more "information," the dissemination of which seldom equates directly with widespread physician compliance or improvements in clinical practice.[13] On the other, to lay heaviest responsibility for the success of EBM on the performance of the individual health professional alone, given his or her obvious cognitive limitations, misses the larger barrier and the larger opportunity. The much-remarked "voltage drop" that occurs in the transmission of medical knowledge down the line from discovery to the laboriously and expensively-trained brains of doctors who are then expected to apply it to sick people, is simply a given of the world we live in. And as discovery accelerates, the "voltage drop" will only get worse.[14]

Failure of health care in America to deliver service that is efficient, patient centered, safe, timely, and so forth indeed owes much to a failure to use best evidence well and consistently. But that is not primarily because of the failure of individual health care workers or even the resistance of doctors protective of their professional autonomy. The larger, and determinative, problem lies with how the overall system of actions and events, all the procedural matrices of health care delivery, work or don't work to enable EBM to deliver on its promise. For all the scientific content of the most definitive clinical practice guideline, it is workaday *procedures*—the way things are done, the habits and structures of the work itself, the conditions in which medical work happens—that in the end cripple or advance the practice of evidence-based medicine.*

The spread of EBM has been made possible both by the realization that something must be done to collect and filter useful information, and by the development of new techniques and tools to do that job.[15] Everyday need for valid information about diagnosis, prognosis, and therapy rises with spiraling expectations placed upon the health care system and presumptions, right or wrong, about the progress of biomedical discovery. Traditional means for meeting this need grow ever less adequate: Textbooks are instantly out of date, the best experts are not infrequently wrong, continuing medical education is typically ineffective, journal literature is simply overwhelming and unreliable. While the doctor's diagnostic skills and clinical judgment typically sharpen with experience, his familiarity with advanced research and findings declines. Rare is the full-time clinician with more than a few seconds to devote, per patient, to finding and assimilating best evidence, to say nothing of time for more general reading.

But tools have been developed to turn this situation around and make possible, and practical, what once was not: mathematical models, decision trees, Bayes' theorem for analyzing diagnostic tests, clinical epidemiology, technology assessment, and meta-analysis.[16] Strategies have been developed for locating and weighing evidence for its validity and relevance. Systematic reviews and distilled summaries of the effects of interventions now exist in abundance. Evidence-based journals whittle down the broader literature to the 2 percent of clinical articles that are both valid and of immediate clinical use. Before digitization, cheap computing and a navigable Internet, this was all largely fanciful. Now, it is made routine through high-quality "foraging tools" that open up the databases *and* cull them for the right information. Beyond systematic surveys, however, the very best tools are ones that filter out *and* arrange data in a hierarchical order. These tools perform validity assessments and assign levels to different kinds of evidence. They can advise on how to apply information in real-world clinical context. They can screen out disease-oriented research (less desirable) from patient-oriented research outcomes.[17]

Hierarchy of Evidence

Level of Evidence	Cochrane Systematic Reviews	Foraging Tools	Hunting Tools
1, A	Other SRs & Meta-Analyses	Cochrane Database	Essential Evidence + Wiley, Dynamed
	Evidence Guidelines	Clinical Evidence	
	Evidence Summaries	DARE	Wiley
	RCTs Case Cohorts, Control Studies	ACP Journal Club	Dynamed
	Clinical Research Critiques	POEMS	Essential Evidence + Dynamed
	Others Reviews of the Literature	USPSTF	Essential Evidence + Dynamed
	Case Reports, Case Series, Practice Guidelines, etc.	National Guidelines Clearinghouse	Essential Evidence + Dynamed
5, C	Clinical Reference Texts	Textbooks	Essential Evidence + Dynamed
	MEDLINE		

Source: http://med.fsu.edu/userimages/EBMPyramid2008-02-26.gif.

A second graphic in a pyramid shape typically is used to depict this hierarchy of evidence, with quality increasing as one approaches the top. In descending order: systematic reviews and meta-analyses, critically appraised topics, critically appraised individual articles; randomized controlled trials, cohort studies, case-controlled studies and reports, and, at the bottom, background information (noise) and "expert" opinion. The highest level of rigor—the gold standard within the gold standard—is probably the Cochrane Database of Systematic Reviews published by the International Cochrane Collaboration, which employs teams of experts to conduct comprehensive literature reviews and present summaries of findings of the best studies. In parallel, The Agency for Health Care Quality and Research's TRIP (Turning Research Into Practice) database searches evidence-based sources of systematic review, practice guidelines, and critically-appraised topics and articles, as well as NIH's MEDLINE Clinical Queries resource. It is a field rich in acronyms. POEMS—Patient-Oriented Evidence that Matters—is probably, well, the most poetic. Published since 1996, it employs a stringent winnowing process that applies specific criteria for validity and relevance to clinical practice.[18]

Certain as Can Be

Examples illustrating the scope of EBM underscore its self-critical nature and how evidence finds its place within the clinical frame. Improvement, as much as standardization, is its theme. Just because something has always been done, even with reasonable success, does not mean that there is not something better, if not at the core then at the margin. Evidence feeds into practice at different speeds, depending. It resolves uncertainty more than it assures brilliance.

What for instance is the best treatment for Bell's Palsy, a facial affliction caused by damage to a facial nerve? Until recently, no one really knew. Sometimes, patients recover spontaneously, sometimes steroids are prescribed, sometimes in combination with antivirals (this because in some cases there may be a tie to the chicken pox virus). Then, in 2004 a study undertaken by primary care doctors in Scotland asked the question "does early treatment with a steroid or an antiviral drug or both affect the recovery of facial function?"[19] A well-powered, double-blind, randomized trial including a control group yielded the clear conclusion that early treatment with a steroid alone significantly improved the likelihood of complete recovery and that there was no advantage only a cost, in adding-on an antiviral.[20]

Whether patients with bowel conditions can avoid unnecessary colonoscopy yielded to a noninvasive test involving a stool analysis that was evaluated against colonoscopies in multiple studies. A meta-analysis showed the simpler procedure effective in distinguishing those most likely to need colonoscopy for more serious bowel disease. This liberated resources to be used in a more targeted way on patients with disorders like Crohn's disease or colon cancer.[21]

Over a period of twenty years, anesthesiologists have investigated invasive versus noninvasive devices to deliver and monitor oxygen supply during surgery. Traditionally, the job was done using wide needles inserted into major veins, but these also slowed recovery and risked postoperative complications. The disposable esophageal Doppler probe, by contrast, required insertion only into the patient's gullet where it measured blood flow using ultrasound. Progressively larger randomized control trials over two decades established that patients undergoing major or high-risk surgery had fewer complications and left the hospital sooner when the Doppler probe was used. Nor were readmissions or repeat operations any more frequent than with other patients. The guideline stipulating that the Doppler probe should be used in high-risk cases was adopted in 2011.[22]

When Jackie Kennedy gave birth to Patrick Bouvier Kennedy in 1963 in an emergency Caesarean section, the premature baby died two days later from respiratory distress syndrome. That this would not happen today is thanks to work begun later that decade by a young researcher who, working with sheep, observed that steroids reduced breathing problems in newborn lambs. Pediatricians then designed randomized, double blind, controlled clinical trials to test whether steroid injection on women undergoing premature labor would improve the respiratory health of their babies. The results, published in 1972, showed higher survival rates with the steroid injections. Trials over subsequent decades confirmed that antenatal steroids save premature lives and cut the risk of respiratory distress syndrome by half.[23]

Obstetricians, meanwhile, tackled the old problem of how best to deliver breech babies, an area that long lacked consensus. A pioneering study in the early 1990s examined 3,477 healthy, full-term, breech births by elective Caesarian, emergency C-section in labor, and vaginal delivery. It suggested that risk of death during or soon after birth was 1 percent for vaginal delivery, but just

.03 percent for C-section. Large clinical trials across numerous hospitals followed, confirming the earlier study and with the result that Caesarian delivery of breech babies has become the evidence-based standard around the world.[24]

Cancer remains the plague-equivalent of modern times although it too is beginning to yield to discovery. The use of radiation therapy to treat and sometimes cure it is not new, but over the past twenty years, randomized trials have cast light on optimum doses and schedules for particular varieties. Some of the best data thus far is for breast cancer. A large 2008 trial tested the international standard dose (50 Gray in 25 doses over 5 weeks) against alternative higher doses administered over a shorter time. A three-week regimen was revealed to offer equally good tumor control but with fewer side effects and, of course, fewer visits to the hospital. Moreover, with breast cancer accounting for approximately one-third of the workload in many radiology departments, the move to compressed treatment schedules, which was quickly and widely adopted, freed-up capacity for treating more patients.[25]

Some of this is the stuff of headlines. Some is highly esoteric. Some is surprisingly ordinary. Famously, it was through randomized, controlled clinical trials begun in the 1980s that treatments have evolved for AIDS, turning the HIV virus infection from a death sentence into a manageable chronic condition. First, it was observed that a cancer drug also reduced deaths among AIDS patients. Next, a combination of three antiretrovirals was then shown to be even more efficacious. Tests for when to begin drug therapy, when and how to adjust it during the clinical course of the disease, and how to manage side effects all ensued. Tests also showed that the right mix of antiretrovirals can stop the spread of the disease from an infected mother to her baby.[26] Exotically, trials have demonstrated how victims of intraocular melanoma can avoid unnecessary screening for spread of cancer to the liver via testing for a particular genetic abnormality (the complete or partial loss of a chromosome 3), which determines whether a patient suffers from the fatal variety of the tumor.[27] Finally, not everything is high-powered science. Evidence-based techniques have been applied to one of the remaining gaping holes in the treatment of heart disease: the fact that many coronary patients (about one-quarter) simply fail to take their anti-clotting medicine just a week after leaving the hospital. This reduces the effectiveness of treatment and increases mortality. Reasons include fear of side effects, the perception that the medication isn't necessary, and, yes, just plain forgetfulness. Evidence shows that support efforts, which can be as simple as reminder cards explaining in lay language the importance of anti-clotting drugs, reiterating the correct dosage, and that the medication should be taken in combination with aspirin, improve patient observance of drug regimens and so broader health outcomes.[28]

Evidence + Expertise

"Is it true?" "Is it useful now?" These are the two questions that EBM in all its iterations aims to answer correctly, every time and in time. The two questions link the two halves of the evidence-based concept. In the evidence-based world, science as represented by the best available external evidence derived from systematic research, reveals truth as biomedical science reveals it. Only individual clinical expertise however—"the proficiency and judgment that individual clinicians acquire through clinical experience and clinical practice"—determines usefulness and fitness for individual patients. Practicing EBM means integrating best evidence with clinical expertise: good science applied *scientifically* to medicine. Neither alone is sufficient; indeed either alone can be dangerous. Balance is everything: in the absence of clinical expertise, "practice risks becoming tyrannized by evidence" (the "cookbook" specter). Yet without searching and applying best evidence, practice cannot possibly stay up-to-date.[29]

Thus epidemiologist David Sackett, one of EBM's founders, defended the movement in 1996 against anonymous critics who accused believers like himself of naïve empiricism, complaining that EBM was "impossible to practice, cookbook medicine, the creature of managers and purchasers, concerned only with randomized trials."[30] More nuanced criticism persists nearly two decades, and many more successes, later (see above). But in fact such criticism has raised few issues that EBM, properly understood, does not accommodate. Such "dissonance" as there may be between the "science" of evidence and the "art" of clinical judgment is muted by EBM's modest (truth be known) intentions from the beginning: To see that treatments used in clinical practice were in fact justified through evidence and that such evidence was rendered accessible to real-world clinicians. EBM does not deny the place of clinical experience and reasoning from basic science. But it does chasten, discipline. And. yes, sometimes correct it: "Instead of having to face the dishearteningly subjective task of basing their decision on intuition we could not explain," Sackett notes, "clinicians had available to them a science that generated objective knowledge of effective interventions based, where possible, on the results of unbiased experiments."[31]

Place remains, perhaps more crucial than ever given new emphasis on patients' participation in their own care, for so-called "narrative-based medicine" in the evidence-based world.[32] A "Campaign for real evidence-based medicine," launched in the summer of 2014 as collaboration between Queen Mary University in London and the University of Oxford's Centre for Evidence Based Medicine, therefore comes as no real surprise and promises an enriched expression of EBM.[33] In the spirit of making a good thing even better, concern for patient-centeredness only recognizes the definitional limits of randomized controlled trials in the first place. Employed in the pursuit of much sought-after truths, randomized trials trade on an acknowledged but important fiction. They depict mainstream "average patients"—who, in the singular form in real practice, do not exist.[34] Every patient is unique and experiences illness in a private context unlike the experience of someone else suffering with the same disease. Evidence-based medicine, at its refined best, presupposes, and in no way dismisses, this reality.[35] Nor, on the other hand, should personal anecdote or "interpreted narrative" be allowed to upend the definitive authority of the randomized clinical trial as arbiter of what most likely works most of the time for most patients. Alertness is everything, and they are poor clinicians who do not interpret what they observe, figuratively and literally, "at the bedside." Increasingly, however, that will be seen as partial text only, which must be fit into the governing context of EBM. With a good fit, the result is optimum—never perfect but optimum—integrated clinical decision-making.

Objective evaluation, let alone precise measurement, of clinical practice has long been elusive. EBM, with its coherent scientific approach to decision making and emphasis on whether interventions actually work in practice, makes measurement and therefore accountability possible. EBM is not the perfect solution; obviously, it is not competent outside the scope of biomedicine. For example, what are the impacts of culture, politics, economics on illness and therapeutics? But EBM does not have to be perfect in order to discipline the practice of medicine for a new system of service and to help narrow the gap between the best of what we know and how we then act upon that knowledge. Indeed, it already has begun to do this very thing.

THREE

Teams Work

For the word *team* one searches the 1910 Flexner Report in vain—and, likewise, the glossary of the medical profession for much of the century following its publication. Flexner's model for making medical doctors fixed on the opposite of *team*: the individual and, as it turned out, the generally autonomous scientific doctor. Such doctors would become the top rank of a newly elite profession founded on inductive science and clinical authority.[1] Flexner was keen to embed medical education into an institutional setting—the research university—where, in the early twentieth century (as, still, in the early twenty-first), *team* primarily conjured up images not from medicine at all but from the world of sports. And in athletics, where competition is everything, the word seldom appears shorn of one of two critical modifiers: *winning* or *losing*.

Such commonplace usages matter. They define the sorts of endeavors, and the purposes served, for which the team—a collective of persons voluntarily associated together in a particular work and who subordinate personal importance for the success of the whole—is deemed the relevant instrument. The young learn team play and team sports in school, both to provide entertainment for parents, schoolmates, and rivals, but also to absorb attitudes and behaviors believed to be virtuous and applicable in settings beyond the playing fields and on into adult life long after schooldays are past. Not all teams, literally, need be voluntary, or even composed of humans. For most of human history, as older dictionaries attest, *team* referred first to teams of animals put to tasks of plowing or hauling. To act as one, they required a harness and the command (and sometimes the lash) of a driver.

In American civic culture, children learn about teams slowly, even as they grow up and develop as individuals. Only-children may be at a disadvantage;

those from large families may get the idea sooner. Gradually, they all learn how self-reliance *teams* (to use the verb form) with reliance on others, in some division of labor, to accomplish the larger task for the larger good. Marriage itself is often spoken of as a *team* endeavor, in which one-plus-one at the altar becomes somehow more than two for a lifetime, where two partners together accomplish more than the same two individuals apart. Outside the home, countless organizations like the scouts, summer camps, organized athletics, school itself extend the awareness of and commitment to the importance of *teamwork* as a routine part of growing up. "Pull together now or fail separately" is drummed into the hardest of youthful heads. Military recruits soon learn to suborn individuality to group identity as well as the imperative of functioning effectively with others in order to achieve the mission. All for one and one for all.

In business culture, teams are commonplace, although their importance was latent until recent times. The history of the firm is, at its base, the history of organizations of individuals configured in various ways to accomplish certain tasks toward desired business goals. Formal study of the role of the team within the larger organization however is relatively new, though it now enjoys a large and respected literature.[2] Companies large and small, faced with tasks where multiple skills and experience must be joined to commitment and accountability, strive to improve performance by cultivating a culture of teams and constantly honing their effectiveness. The mid-twentieth century cliché of the "organization man [and men] in the gray flannel suit" gives way to that of the multidisciplinary, multi-skilled, multi-experienced, diverse team, to say nothing of new understandings of the role of leadership, performance challenges, and the nature of accountability.

Legacy

In the cultures of medicine and health care, teams by comparison feel like foreign bodies. Whereas the notion of teams and teamwork evolves naturally in family and civic life and has taken the corporate and management world more or less by storm, its impact in health care has proven tentative at best. Although one of the largest and most complex "industries" in America, health care lags far behind when it comes to organizing its talent to achieve its mission.

Two factors primarily account for, if not excuse, this fact. One is environmental, embedded deep within the economic structure and professional creeds of the business of medicine as it has grown up in the twentieth century. Of course, there are organizational exceptions—the relatively controlled environments of large academic health centers and the exceptional instances outside academe like Kaiser Permanente and Intermountain Health Care. Though transition is evident, most health care as it is currently dispensed remains small scale, proudly independent and financed on the fee-for-service principle. It shares this with other professions granted quasi-monopoly rights in return for maintenance of high ethical standards and some element of public service. The solo or small specialty group practice is where most doctors still find employment and professional fulfillment, and it is an experience that does not predispose them positively toward teams. Moreover, the process of professionalization as it has occurred in medicine, with its relentless emphasis on the role of the credentialed expert and the sanctity of that one individual's relationship with patients, further retards the sharing of responsibility and authority with other levels of health care providers.

The second factor accounting for the relative rarity of teams in health care is educational. Medical schools today remain remarkably faithful to the Flexnerian reforms that aimed to unify science and medicine a century ago. Those reforms succeeded wonderfully but at some cost. That they happened quickly was due to a beneficent confluence of interests and resources, but they also evolved through the decades. As they did so, and as more and more schools sprouted to supply the personnel needed to meet increasing demand for the wonders of modern medicine, consensus about the identity and character of those personnel seldom wavered. Medical schools trained, first and above all, scientifically literate and clinically experienced individual MDs and, as time passed, increasingly specialized ones. On them as *individuals*, fierce training bestowed the authority that flows from the ability to take responsibility for others. Nothing in that experience said anything about cooperation or working collaboratively with other sorts of professionals, although many doctors obviously did so to varying degrees. Medicine remained a profession of and for accomplished individuals.[3]

In one sense however there was about medical education an even older bias toward individual autonomy that Flexner only reinforced. Since the "heroic" days of the nineteenth century and before, doctors-to-be had learned the little they then knew primarily by apprenticeship: by watching, listening, following, copying the example of those who had learned and done medicine before them. Apprentices learned, and learn, from masters, one on one. Flexner did not fundamentally change this form of teaching and learning. What he added was structure, content and resources. The resulting model was, and remains, a pedagogy that is intensely personal not corporate.

Taken together, the enduring, fractured structure of medical provision and the formation of medical doctors primarily as autonomous actors from their first encounters with the educational process have conspired to keep the idea of teams in the background. This persists even now and just when science, which has lifted medicine to heights unimagined by Flexner's generation, approaches a crisis of service that cannot be met other than by teams.

In what was to become the *ur*-text of team performance in the management and business worlds, Jon R. Katzenbach and Douglas K. Smith's *The Wisdom of Teams: Creating the High-Performance Organization*, the teams researched ranged widely, from a high school basketball team to the US Army to a major management consulting firm to numerous *FORTUNE* 1000 companies to the Girl Scouts. With the exception of one pharmaceutical company, no teams from health care organizations made the list. Neither "medicine" nor "health care" appears in the index. Published in 1993, *The Wisdom of Teams* was the work of respected management consultants—both Katzenbach and Smith had worked at the venerable McKinsey & Company—but it would be a decade and more before the message would take hold in health care. Those making the case there, although no longer voices in the wilderness, still faced an uphill climb.[4]

Moreover, even as examples accumulated of teams' superior care particularly in the management of chronic disease, the problem was that the evidence remained at the margin. This is not to dismiss it as in any way marginal for those personally involved, either as providers or patients. Lives have been saved, suffering eased, health restored, costs cut. It is however to make the distinction between organizational change that is bolted-on to an existing regime of provision, and cultural change that is built-in at the very beginning of an entirely new system of provision. The power of the former to effect further change is the limited power of example: A message that insists that "here, you too can copy this behavior and if you do you will achieve these kinds of results." Its power is no greater and no less than the power of any option that offers the opportunity of a choice without being able to compel the right one. The power of the latter, of change that is built-in and constitutional to a system, is of a different order of magnitude entirely. It not only presumes a fresh start but also, progressing ahead, brooks no alternative. It commands—either emulation or dismissal.

Until a culture of teams in health care is planted at the level of educational inputs, the organization of teams in health care will continue largely ad hoc, dependent on exceptional leadership and fortuitous circumstance. Instances where this union has occurred demonstrate the possibilities, even if they do not yet radically alter the probabilities.

Exemplar

Nowhere have leadership and circumstance converged with quite the effect and on quite the scale as at Kaiser Permanente. This of course is anomalous because Kaiser, in an American context, is anomalous. An independently owned, integrated health services delivery company, with its own insurance plan and wholly salaried medical staff, it lies far off the beaten path of the American experience, and it is not likely to become the main highway any time soon. Extreme examples can however cast sharp light at least on the probable path ahead, even if not quite all the way to the final goal. Such is the usefulness of Kaiser.

The team approach to care delivery evolved at Kaiser more as a response to particular circumstances than as the result of grand strategy. Rudiments began to appear in the 1960s, first with the introduction of efforts to undertake significant front-end screening and counseling for the "worried well."[5] Sidney R. Garfield, Kaiser physician and keen observer of the distinction between "sick care" and "health care," was also notable in pushing the notion of a team-based approach to such screening and campaigned hard for development of screening centers through the 1970s. There was no formal, top-down policy. What occurred, however, occurred in a particular context, with a combination of supportive incentives resulting from global capitation and the forced togetherness that occurs in an integrated multispecialty delivery system like Kaiser. Probably the single most telling factor was that "togetherness" happened not only among physicians, but also with nurses and varieties of other health professionals in the clinical setting. Gradually it became clear, based first on the quality of the day-to-day clinical experience and later in the measureable long-term results, that working collaboratively made more sense that hewing to the traditional model of the isolated, autonomous physician in lordly relationship with "his or "her" patient.

The realization crystalized fastest in settings where children were involved, asthmatics especially, or where a high level of education and support were required generally, as with diabetics. With chronic diseases, it was clear quite early that if patients could be taught to live healthier lives, and convinced to sustain better habits, that complications and preventable mortality would decline. What in essence happened was that the coalescence of teams at Kaiser followed a path of least resistance, where the limits of classic physician-centric practice were most obvious, and where the availability of resources made it possible for informal teams to develop. "A process of demonstration and example," Kaiser CEO Emeritus David Lawrence modestly called it.[6]

The one exception to this *ad hoc* dynamic, which was driven largely from inside the clinic, arose from Kaiser's fraught relationship with its unions and the labor unrest of the 1980s and 1990s.[7] The upshot of the agreement reached between David Lawrence and John Sweeney was a formal labor-management partnership, still in effect, which today covers twenty-five of the thirty-six unions at Kaiser Permanente and more than 80 percent of the represented workforce. Although it excluded the California Nurses Association, which never joined the partnership, the influence of the partnership changed profoundly the way all unions work with management. At the core of the new regime lay agreement that both sides needed to work collaboratively and in teams to solve a wide range of problems in the institution, ranging from conditions of work, safety for workers, and of course at the core purpose of the organization: patient care.

Care at Kaiser has come to mean care in teams and nothing else. "Care teams," not "doctors and nurses," are what deliver care. It sounds like a tautology but isn't. Kaiser's David Lawrence may be the single most dedicated evangelist for the centrality of the care team concept as the best hope for meeting the challenges that beset the practice of medicine and the delivery of health care.[8] Without it, none of the Institute of Medicine's expansive goals for the health care system stand any lasting chance of achievement.[9] This failure, it is important to note, has little if anything to do with competence. Most health care professionals in America today, from the newly graduated to the most senior, are well-trained, conscientious, best-intentioned individuals. Many, probably a large majority, will say the reason they went into medicine in the first place was to "help people" or "make a difference in the world." (The fact that many have made good livings and even grown wealthy along the way should not impugn their noble motives.) In medicine, for decades in America at least, it was widely accepted that doing well and doing good worked nicely enough in tandem. On the supply side, providers prospered as demand for care rose. On the demand side, the vast majority of the cared-for benefited from ample supply of services and high levels of technical expertise. However, the very thing that enabled the endless "advance of medical science"—research that explained more of the puzzles and led to better clinical solutions—also frustrated its delivery. As individual doctor's knowledge inevitably became deeper than it was broad, it became a cliché that specialism was inimical to caring for the "whole person." The "primary care" that most people need first and most of the time was presumed to be fundamentally at odds with specialism. However true, this was unhelpful. Specialization was not about to end unless science ended, and science, as the past century of medical advance showed, was what made the whole ship go. If in this respect alone, health care's future is likely to track medicine's past.

The frustration among the cared-for arose because medical advance yielded complexity rather than simplicity. The more complex, or long-lasting, one's affliction, the larger the number of people one's care would involve. Chronic disease was to the early twenty-first century what infectious disease was to the early twentieth, and it has proved as yet susceptible to few solutions equivalent in their elegant simplicity to penicillin and polio vaccine. What most baffles sick people (the worried well among them) today is that when they get sick and present themselves to their doctor, thereafter they too soon stand a good chance of getting lost in the maze of the system, which is itself what J. D. Kleinke has termed an "oxymoron."[10] The sicker one is, or the longer one remains sick, the greater the number of health care providers one needs. These good people belong, at best, to a loose federation, allied in the general purpose of healing but hampered by bad business models, poorly trained, and inadequately incentivized for the coordination and communication needed to accomplish their noble purpose.

For the vast majority of Americans who do not enjoy access to Kaiser and a select few other integrated care providers like it, and who consequently must navigate medicine's maze as best they can, the care team concept offers hope to overcoming the huge obstacle to quality delivery. To the twin demons of fragmentation and lack of continuity in care, which together block the path of translation of the best science in medicine into delivery of the best health care, teams are the fundamental structural answer.

David Lawrence speaks of care teams with emotion, as the place where the "human relationships at the heart of medicine occur."[11] They are the place where the patient is invited to seek and to find care most appropriate to his unique needs and then to participate with medical professionals in his care or hopefully his cure. It is at the beginning point, or at this core, that old notions of patient care first caused doctors to stumble. As when Cornwallis surrendered at Yorktown in 1781 and the world turned upside down (here, perhaps, inside out), it is as if the patient and not the physician constitutes the center of the team in the new dispensation. Coalesced around the patient— as a person and a participant not as a host for disease and the passive subject for its attempted cure—the team exists to provide two elements most critical to care: the skills of highly trained individual professionals *plus* the networks of relationships through which that knowledge and those skills translate into care that is coordinated, consistent, and in keeping with the evidence from the science of what works best—put simply, care that is safe and of high quality.

Who and How?

The notion of teams applies with equal ease to any number of settings. Teams may be for primary care itself. They may focus on special pathologies from asthma to renal failure to diabetes to heart and vascular disorder. They may have to do with prevention issues, as for screening for prostate, colorectal, or breast cancer. Health maintenance matters may also be the focus, for the healthy elderly or for youth.

Different sets of individuals may constitute different sorts of teams depending on the subject, yet they will share common membership in the team. Doctors are key to all teams, although they are not necessarily central or even necessarily leaders. "My doctor" is a cozy notion, which implies personal physician/patient relationship that is in fact very difficult to achieve and sustain in modern practice settings, even at the level of primary care. Honesty at least requires some different phrasing. In team settings, there may well be other physicians besides one's "primary" doctor and whose role may, as needs be, supercede that individual. A nurse care manager likely fills essential multiple, border-crossing roles, not the least of which is the coordination of care within a team. Any variety of other professionals will fill out a team, from nurse practitioners (employed not merely as labor-savors for physicians but also as skilled clinicians in their own right best deployed at the frontlines of the care process), to pharmacists, nutritionists, social workers, and educators.

Teams function not by happenstance but because they are designed and built to do so, according to carefully worked out and scrupulously observed principles and standards of behavior. They do not come about without perseverance, and they do not last without constant maintenance. New skills must be acquired and practiced until they become habit.[12] Above all, the sharing of information and the sharing of decision making must become first-nature. As the need for continuing professional education at the individual level is universally understood, so too is the need for continuing team nourishment. Teams must be able to define team leadership and identify a team leader (not necessarily a physician) and establish care guidelines that include the patient as an equal, even central, participant in the care process. They must learn to communicate ceaselessly; they must be able to harvest new knowledge as it becomes available from medical research in order both to optimize treatment now and to measure and improve collective performance in the future.

None of this is possible without adoption of electronic information and knowledge management systems to collect data and keep evidence current. And because teams are not invulnerable to the very sort of isolation that bedevils care delivery by solo practitioners and single-specialty practices, the success of teams presupposes the support of larger external organizations that can provide scale and link teams to one another and to non-medical resources in communities. And bridges must be built to the community itself, through public health departments, consumer advocacy groups, and disease-specific organizations (from AARP to Families USA to the American Cancer Society to the Epilepsy Foundation). Even alternative providers, osteopathic physicians for example, once-dismissed to the shady margins of medicine's well-guarded territory, have been known to function happily on the same team with conventional care-givers.[13]

Health care, it is increasingly said, is a team sport, and those who are not collaborative by nature or even trainable as team players might perhaps look elsewhere for professional satisfaction. The trouble is that the health care profession is filled already with people without such formative training and some with actual hostility toward the whole concept of integrated team care. The concept is not utterly new—certainly, it is less new than the digitization of medical re-cords, the benefits of which seem obvious but whose adoption remains equal-ly slow. The Mayo Clinic, founded over a century ago and before the craft/physician-centric model of health care delivery achieved the dominance it still enjoys, from the very start practiced according to team-integrated delivery prin-ciples and never felt much need to talk about it. Today at Mayo, it remains more assumed than asserted. The Kaiser system, which enrolls more than 8 mil-lion individuals is the single largest exemplar of the team principle, extended to integrate financing as well as delivery systems. Health Partners in Boston and the Henry Ford Health System stand out as similarly effective team-driven organizations. Cleveland Clinic and Virginia Mason Clinic in Seattle have been working at it with steady improvement for several decades. Other instances, like the MD Anderson Cancer Center, Sloan Kettering, and the National Jewish Hospital for Children, demonstrate the principle applied in specialty settings.[14]

David Lawrence argues that only in such integrated team-based care lies any hope of meeting the tangle of challenges bearing down on health care delivery in the century to come: from daunting patient expectations (for both right results and to be active rather than passive players in a transparent care process), to the growing prevalence of chronic disease that can as yet only be managed not cured, to the complexity of care and the information explosion brought on by biomedi-cal discovery. To this challenge and the integrated team-based solution, the ques-tion of how care is paid for—literally of who "owns" it, as in the private sector or the state—may not in fact be the central one. In Britain's wholly government-fi-nanced, free-to-all-at-point-of-service, GP-centric National Health Service, the fragmentation of care is little different from what it is in the United States, where with some exceptions (admittedly very large ones: the Veterans Administration, Medicare/Medicaid, government employees, the active-serving military, and the Indian Health Service) care is financed through a bedlam of private insurance schemes. A central question is, however, how to reconcile the widespread desire that most patients have for a primary relationship with "their physician," a desire enforced by law and custom, with the requirements of team-based-care where physicians share authority in the context of collective knowledge. Technology races ahead here, with its demand for mastery of more information than any sin-gle doctor can ever manage and without which it becomes impossible to practice competently or even safely. Nostalgia among those readers of a certain age for the doctors of their childhoods, who made house calls, often at odd hours, and who carried everything they could need in their little black bags, lives on hazardously into an era when the volume and velocity of science overwhelms the most brilliant paragons of a profession habituated to their own authority and autonomy.

The Blender

Although integrated team-based care remains the exception in American health care delivery, examples grow, as above, of the concept's success at high institutional level. Wherever it is practiced in earnest and with persistence, it delivers improved outcomes for patients and providers alike. Why exactly this is so may be observed best however at a lower altitude, in small laboratories of teamwork which, while unique in some of their founding circumstances, are nonetheless replicable elsewhere, whether inside the most rarefied academic settings or back home on Main Street.

Teams are the device whereby care can be blended among specialties. Science dictates specialization in research, which, if it is to translate broadly, must be blended ("de-specialized") in practice. This insight as yet has no home in medical education and comes about most often on the job, among patients, who need care but who should not be burdened with the responsibility to find it. Patients encounter medicine's specialization early and experience it endlessly, and they know the countervailing truth that everything overlaps whatever the sign says on the clinic or the doctor's door. They know, first, that there are so-called physicians who diagnose and then prescribe medications and other treatments, and that there are surgeons who operate. Often patients need both: "The medicine is no longer working, and so surgery is indicated, … or surgery is not what they need but more or different medicine." In the absence of teams, a natural tendency to satisfy this problem seldom results in true collaboration but in lateral passing back-and-forth of patients between physicians and surgeons and other specialists. From where the patient stands, the experience of such hand-offs is seldom seamless.

The founder of the integrated team-based clinic used for illustration here, Vanderbilt's Asthma Sinus Allergy Program (ASAP), first came to a revelation about teams opportunistically and with common sense.[15] Qualified in both rheumatology and allergy, Simpson B. "Bobo" Tanner had partnered with an orthopedic surgeon specializing in hip and knee replacements and who was interested in bringing rheumatology into a practice centered on arthritis. An arthritis center resulted, called just that because that was what patients, whose joints hurt, supposed they had. They needed a place to go for that affliction and where the professionals—physical therapists, hand therapists, rheumatologists, and orthopedic joint replacement surgeons—would sort out whether or not they needed medical care, surgical care, physical therapy, or a combination. The team concept at that point developed *ad hoc*, but the realization dawned early (and proved permanent) that the face given to the public for what was on offer should also be a face meant for patients, not doctors. "Orthopedics," "rheumatology," "immunology" describe arcane specialties derived from the world of science, not suffering. Joint pain, to sufferers, meant "arthritis," and so would read the name on the new shingle. "We all like to dress up our titles," Tanner admits of the profession. "But frankly, patients would rather not hear the word *otolaryngology*. They want to know whom to go to when they have a problem with their ears, noses and throats."[16]

To name the problem and not the science, which may or may not solve the problem, is to communicate the singular nature of the task at hand, which is to deliver health care to patients. To name, instead, the medical specialties involved in delivering that care would have communicated a different focus, one on doctors and science. To name the problem declared that whatever happened inside those doors would be patient-centered, first to last. This was no cliché. Patient-centered in this particular circumstance meant integrated care among specialties and levels of care provider. Integrated care meant teams. Therefore: Advertise the problem—the reason care is necessary—and not the scientific nomenclature for possible solutions to it.

To blend medical specialties together in dynamic delivery settings requires steady leadership and considerable cross-cultural learning. Before Tanner's center was established, separate clinics had coordinated events haphazardly at best. Patients with sinus problems might be sent to surgeons or for lung tests, then wait several days for results to return before having skin tests. There was no shortage of inefficiencies for everyone involved. Patients had to arrange time off from work to meet different appointments on different days. For care providers, often physically separated and untrained in teamwork, the process of diagnosis and development of a coherent treatment plan could take an unnecessarily long time. The particular decision at this institution to move ahead with a self-contained, integrated center for asthma, sinus, and allergy was initially top-down and unique to the leadership then at hand, but the ensuing experience with blended practice over the long term suggested elements that were not unique. The decision for integration required two critical tools: electronic medical records capability (which at first had to be outsourced) and the use of nurse practitioners in new ways.

Nurse practitioners, of which the local nursing school graduated some 150 each year, were most commonly deployed in primary care settings where they were seen to extend physicians' reach. ASAP, however, used then in a blended specialty setting where they would serve in another function and meet other needs altogether. These had to do with discoveries about how best to match up patients' expectations with doctors' talents. Experience in the Arthritis Center had shown something of an 80–20 needs ratio, with 80 percent of patients needing relatively routine care and 20 percent something more extended and exotic. The problem was that the sorting-out often occurred on the surgeon's doorstep, a late and wasteful point for most patients, and even more so for the surgeons who ended up seeing too many patients who didn't need a surgeon at all. ASAP changed all this. A sinus surgeon could walk into the waiting room in the morning assured that all, or very close to all, of those patients who were to see him actually needed his skills—because they had passed a filter and been cleared.

With not enough allergist MDs to go around, the filter became the nurse-practitioner equipped with a set of precise standardized tools. The concept could stir suspicions. Referring community physicians sometimes feared that their patients would never be able to see the high-powered MD specialist at all. To academic doctors at research-oriented tertiary-care AHCs, the practice could smack of downright betrayal of historic mission: the conviction that each patient is unique and each doctor-patient relationship equally so, and that nothing can be allowed to come between them. It is not unlike the allure of the custom-built house, when in fact a house built from standardized plans suits most people—and budgets—well enough.

The nurse practitioner strategy also attacked the problem at the point where most patients experience their first frustration with the system, that is, the speed of access. When ASAP was just starting, a three-month wait to see an allergy specialist was not uncommon. Sinus surgeons were seeing patients they didn't need to see, who needed medical not surgical treatment. Delivery of medical treatment was disjointed, inconvenient, and inevitably inconsistent.

Two things were required to equip generalist nurse practitioners to improve this kind of experience: evidence-based protocols to follow with each and every patient, and electronic records with a questionnaire that used patients' answers to indicate the next steps in the process. Some patients clearly needed a chest x-ray; some didn't. Some needed allergy testing; some didn't. The compilation of questions was carefully designed to assure that the nurse practitioner could leave nothing out, and the electronic record provided the necessary signposts for further guidance. The evidence base eventually evolved, collaboratively through many meetings and endless questions: "What do we really know? Why do we know that steroids really help people with sinus infections, and what is the data? How long do we treat: two weeks or three? And what do we really *not* know yet?" This was fertile ground for clinical studies using the center's own experience, and it opened new doors for nurse practitioners to participate in the generation of new knowledge rather than just carry out orders. Nurses became able to say, for instance, based on X number of patients over Y period, that intravenous antibiotics used on hard-to-treat sinus infections yielded no better results that those taken orally.

Evidence-based protocols enabled improved process: literally, better patient flow-through. Under the old model, a patient came in to see, at the beginning, the doctor for an initial evaluation. If he said, "yes, you probably have allergies," then the patient might be scheduled to return the following week for skin testing, after which another visit was needed to talk over the results. If the patient also complained of a cough, she might be sent for a chest x-ray, which required *another* meeting to go over those results. In fact, the real problem might really be asthma. To chase that down, a pulmonary function test would be ordered, which required another meeting to go over still more results. It was an incredibly dense process, a not-quite-random but at best loosely linked series of events.

The new aim, and what became a whole new model, was a bit different. A visit remained long (3 to 4 hours), but it became just that: one visit on one day, and it was a full and active day. Condensed, the goal was to sign in, go through the battery of protocol questions in an exam conducted by a nurse practitioner and then, based on the protocol outcomes, proceed to the tests indicated, all of which were available onsite. An appointment consisted actually of two appointments booked on the same day, the initial one with the nurse practitioner for 30 to 45 minutes, followed by the indicated testing regimen, followed by another consultation based on the test results when the physician would also be called in, fully informed. "We were able to get patients to come in, spend four hours and essentially get five or six different visits compressed into one," Simpson recalls. "We went through the whole system, and instead of a six-week to three-month waiting list, we got it down to two weeks."[17]

Although the physician's role was later in the process, it was intensified. At the concluding consultation, with the patient present along with family and the nurse practitioner (who thenceforth remains primary contact), the physician reviews the test findings: "This is your sinus CT scan that showed a sinus infection on the left and here is the picture showing the problem and explaining the anatomy." This is hugely different from calling a patient and reading the disembodied results over the phone. The physician may then do a more focused exam just to clarify some pieces of the picture and perhaps ask some additional, off-protocol questions. Then, a written treatment plan is presented for the patient to consider—where we're going, what the next steps are, and what everyone can expect. The physician was always available, although with the eighty percent of cases that are fairly routine, usually not present until the conference at visit's end. On follow-up visits, if called for, nurse practitioners on their own managed their patients unless a new problem had appeared, at which point, a doctor would again be summoned.

In contrast to other models that applied talent scattershot, this systematized, dynamic division of labor had rewarding consequences for doctors as well. Excessively ordinary cases bore highly-trained specialists, who use their training and experience best when challenged most. "You've got to put on your thinking cap on and dig deep," Tanner put it. "When they call you into the room at the end of a visit, or if they call to say they suspect something unusual, you've got to be ready for some real challenges. It isn't ho-hum."[18] It is the nurse practitioners, however, who give the team its unique participatory flavor and drive home the virtues of team care for patients. Nurse practitioners come from a background of teaching, and thrive on showing patients how to do things. Physicians are not, as a group, famously good at this; nurse practitioners do it willingly and well. Nurse practitioners teach patients what they can and must do to take responsibility for their own care, for seeing they understand the reason for their condition and have the tools to ameliorate it to the degree possible. To employ them on the front-end of the team-care process, not as mere doctor-extenders randomly along the way (or in hospital settings as glorified RNs), was key to ASAP's integrated approach to care. Nurse practitioners communicated by temperament, probably better than most doctors, that the patient arriving at the clinic each morning would in fact be *cared for*, if not cured, although sometimes that too. Patients immediately warmed to their presence, and complaints of "only wanting to see a doctor" were almost never heard. What was enormously satisfying for patients was also satisfying for the professionals who cared for them first and continuously.

It was of course challenging to nurse practitioners to find themselves on the frontlines of medical decision-making. Tethered to evidence-based protocols, nurse practitioners were called on to take responsibility disproportionate, skeptics would say, to their training. This perception proved not just unkind but inaccurate. To be challenged is to experience the opportunity to grow. ASAP's corps of nurse practitioners would grow steadily in numbers, in competence, and in self-confidence, and while not physicians, within a few years of working within a specialty they become experts at treating discrete disease processes. In the context of the team approach, they also have the advantage of being able to spend on each patient more of that most precious of all health care commodities: time. As mid-level providers, they are paid less than physicians and therefore can afford to see fewer patients in a day and spend more time with them. This is the second of two revolutions in the handling of time. The first is radically shortening the time it takes to get an appointment. The second is lengthening the time that a patient routinely spends in face-to-face consultation with health care professionals. Chief of these is the nurse practitioner.

Susan Ficken, lead nurse practitioner at ASAP for a dozen years, speaks directly about techniques for putting patients at ease from the very start, by being sure they know the shape of their visit to come and what exactly to expect. Patients are told ahead of time that their appointment will last three to four hours and that they can "bring a book if they want but that they will be pretty busy." With a light touch but a true one, she tells patients in the initial meeting, "I'm trying to keep you away from the surgeon."[19] They are in for aggressive medical management, which also suits the surgeons. Ficken orchestrates a drill that is personalized but standardized. After paperwork at the front desk, a nurse takes vital signs and prepares the patient to see the nurse practitioner. Most patients, being referred from outside the program, come without extensive records and almost never electronic ones: "We just take a fresh look at them and start over," says Ficken. The nurse practitioner obtains a detailed history and physical, notes current medications, and then decides what needs to be done that day. If a sinus or upper airway situation is indicated, probably only allergy tests are called for, plus perhaps a sinus scan. If there are lower airway problems, chest x-rays and pulmonary function tests will go on the agenda, too. The test regimen is driven by what the history and the physical shows.

Testing proceeds directly and without delay, in dedicated facilities one floor below. Nurses, radiology technicians, respiratory therapists take patients through their pre-scripted regimens, with results entered immediately into the patient's newly created electronic record. Patients then begin an education program tailored to their diagnosis. A certified asthma educator is part of the care team and is in charge of allergy education. Before returning to the nurse practitioner, she will have reviewed the test results and formed an impression, from which a tentative treatment plan takes shape. At the concluding meeting with the patient, test results are reviewed and explained. When the doctor arrives, the nurse practitioner presents the case thus far. The doctor then double-checks and questions further, if need be. The treatment plan is finalized and agreed upon by everyone in the room. The patient is then dispatched home to local physicians. On follow-up visits, if necessary, patients remain primarily under the care of the original nurse practitioners, who enlist physicians only if there is a new problem or if improvement is not proceeding as it should according to the care protocol. Patients with the most challenging problems will require physician attention on every visit, a contingency also built into the system. Territorial possessiveness has no place: "I think that person deserves to get the whole-brain team every time they're here," Ficken notes.[20]

Care thus personalized *and* routinized becomes consistent care. The same responses for the same conditions are delivered in the same ways to different people who are treated as individuals rather than averages—*in spite of the fact that their afflictions can be treated as such*. Such care is talent-intensive but also time-efficient. The patient perceives receiving, and indeed does receive, a lot of time, from an array of focused professionals. Because of the structure of the system, however, the professionals perceive little if any waste of their own time. The system matches their specialized skills with patients' specialized needs. Every medical professional may not yet be temperamentally suited to team medicine—but this is a fact that needs to change. Too few are trained in anticipation of careers spent in structured collaboration with others. It is worth noting that those who do manage to self-sort into settings like ASAP report high levels of job satisfaction.

Nor is America's arcane payment system, which reimburses more for procedures than for delivery of intellectual content, let alone outcomes, particularly friendly to integrated care delivery systems like ASAP. Payers deal with highly structured concepts of how medicine is practiced now, to which blended delivery can look like a disturbing blur. To have patients being seen by several specialists for the same problem on the same day in the same building comports poorly with the old model and requires, from administrators, skilled navigation and negotiation.[21] Creative, yet commonsense, cross-subsidy and revenue-sharing across skills can be necessary. Even if, for instance, it is difficult to determine a discrete fee schedule for the time needed for a nurse to teach a patient how to use nasal sprays and inhalers, there would be enough margin in testing, injections, and scans to cover such activity. All too often, perversely, the pay system seems more like a game of *Battleship* in which one player fires off a salvo without having a clue as to the location of his opponent's ship.

Blended care can be a big stretch for payers looking only at mandated reimbursement categories, but ASAP administrators learned from their experience of hits and misses and gradually refined their aim. The best tactic turned out to be a full-time employee dedicated to calling insurers before a patient arrives to alert them that procedure is anticipated and to request prior authorization. Once it was learned what questions insurers would likely ask, an administrator could back-translate to clinicians (who do not want to delay, because the patient is sitting in the waiting room right now) that a particular test needed to be done in order to get authorization. It is not ideal or inexpensive, but with attentiveness it can be made to work well enough.

Aside from the few large institutional examples like Kaiser, integrated multi-specialty team-based care is most likely to advance near-term in such local settings as ASAP, sometimes at the center, sometimes at the edges of AHCs on whose concentrations of clinical talent, research depth, and information infrastructures they can piggyback. Although they are the primary beneficiaries, patients tend to be more opportunistic than analytical when it comes to choosing such care. It appeals, first and last, because it eases transitions and makes appear seamless and unified what is in fact the complex product of relentlessly advancing specialism. ASAP, as the name suggests, is quick and easy to use. It is part of, yet stands physically apart from, a large medical campus, which like many is a dense stand of towers and connectors daunting to navigate and intimidating for their vast scale alone. ASAP has a building of its own (recycled 1970s-vintage office space), situated unpretentiously between a hotel and a restaurant on a main arterial road just half a mile from a major interstate interchange. Parking is free, abundant and close-at-hand. Patients enter, from back or front, into a pleasant atrium-styled waiting room (better thought of however less as a waiting room, given that nobody ever waits for very long, than as a staging area) where, at multiple front sign-in desks, the care process begins. Most patients come as referrals. A few, particularly at the beginning (and this was a useful lesson), were self-referrals who simply saw the sign out front, or whose friends or relations had had a good experience and recommended it—the "They know what they're doing there and explained it to me," word-of-mouth, sort of marketing. And no one at ASAP hides behind the dreaded "they"—as in "they should have done that test before sending you to me" or "they're always running behind down there." Care comes exclusively in the first-person plural. No one makes professional laterals hard for patients to follow. No one sends a patient scurrying for a record. Everyone plays together and takes responsibility, all the time. Everyone in responsible for outcomes.

A Walk Down the Hall

In another example of team-based care in fields traditionally territorial, outcomes again bear out the virtues of integration.[22] Keith and Andre Churchwell (brothers and colleagues in cardiology at Vanderbilt) like to use the phrase "hybrid care," which means much the same thing as what happens on the far edge of the campus at ASAP. The origins of their Heart and Vascular Institute were both strategic and opportunistic. The home institution was then attempting to crack top-twenty status among AHCs, and to do so it had to have an extremely strong clinical cardiovascular program at its core. This capability might have been acquired as a package and imported from the outside. As it turned out, disgruntlement at a large local competitor made possible recruitment of critical talent close at hand to the Churchwells' vision of integrated heart care, all the while fortifying community goodwill. Since its full consolidation, the resulting institute's example of team-based delivery has changed the image of a research and teaching-oriented institution like many others historically less than revered for the quality of its patient care.

Unlike ASAP, the Heart and Vascular Institute is embedded within the AHC's medical towers, yet is functionally freestanding with its own governance and its own vision of how cardiac care is optimally delivered. At most institutions, and in most communities, cardiovascular medicine is, to borrow from management-speak, practiced in "silos": cardiology, cardiovascular surgery, and vascular surgery. In each, they share the same patient population. Yet hardly anywhere do the doctors talk to each other. "At times they are frankly competitive, which is ultimately destructive of good patient care."[23] This is no longer the case. The change might have been a fortuitous, one-off instance of the happy alignment of particular doctors' ambition and opportunity. But external forces were also at work, which make this one example suggestive as a replicable model for integrated cardiac care elsewhere.

One reason for the change is financial. The days of the large single-specialty group practice, like cardiologists, are likely numbered. Hospital systems vie to make themselves appear attractive partners. One solid attraction is infrastructure costs that have already been met and that can be hard to replicate and sustain at smaller scale. A fully interoperable system of electronic medical records enables physicians and surgeons to work at higher pace even as they work with greater consistency and deliver higher quality. The cost of protecting against malpractice, too, benefits from connectivity. Science and service themselves conspire in the direction of integration because of the increased velocity of the former and the drive for measurement and accountability with the latter. The push for enhanced clinical translation that brings the fruit of discovery more quickly to the practitioner magnifies the importance of the clinician to the AHC because clinicians deliver care—that is, they render service (which is what is paid for)—and deliver it in measureable ways.[24] "Before," as Andre Churchwell bluntly puts it, "it was just grinding up rats and measuring assays." Now, the push for outcomes favors integrated care, which speeds translation. "We can go relatively quickly from some new DNA probe right to the bedside; we need to have people who are smart, active and know how to do that and who want to do clinical research."[25]

Claims to be doing this sort of integrated cardiac care are made in many places. The Churchwells, who visit many such facilities, have an easy way of judging them. When they find few conversations happening, they know not much lasting can be achieved. Team medicine means not endless meetings but endless conversations, some formal and but many more that take place "just walking down the hallway"—true indicators of a culture of collaboration. Anyplace that doesn't have this, that doesn't understand that problem solving is ultimately a group exercise, has not arrived even at the starting point. For a senior surgeon to consult with a senior cardiologist, it is only necessary to walk down the hall to the echo lab and say, "I've got a patient who's got this significant problem; could you walk down the hall so we can have a look together?" The patient, who hears the subsequent dialogue among the experts, is amazed: "So did you just *show up?*" What appears serendipitous from a patient's perspective is in fact built in to the system, a sign of team culture.[26]

Critical Conditions

As care is made consistent, as in integrated team-based settings, quality goes up, safety improves, and price falls. Patients enter the system without fear of losing their way or of being subject, as their particular condition might prompt, to endless professional hand-offs. The professionals learn that their collective efforts, when systematized and made measurable, add up to more than the sum of the parts. Competence increases beyond credentials.

For the time being and to whatever extent it is learned at all, most of this still must be learned by doing, not formally but on the job. This pioneering, experimental spirit is faithful to time-honored traditions of how, for a century, doctors and other health care professionals have learned how to practice what it is they know. First, they fill themselves with knowledge. Then, they serve an apprenticeship. Then, they do it for themselves, perhaps soon even teaching others. For MDs, the process consumes eight to ten years, but still much is left out. Omissions of content are increasingly common but equally understandable, the result of burgeoning biomedical knowledge, but these gaps are manageable through the informatics technology. Omissions of process are another matter. Relatively few medical graduates and those emerging from residency into practice have more than passing acquaintance with the concepts of inter-disciplinary teamwork key to delivery of integrated, patient-centered care. Of the Institute of Medicine's list of core competencies for all health care professions—provision of patient-centered care; ability to work in inter-disciplinary teams; employment of evidence-based medicine; application of quality improvement techniques; use of informatics—the team deficit may still be the most glaring.[27] Filling it, finally, waits upon fixing undergraduate and post-graduate medical education broadly, in ways analogous to how it was improved a century ago following the Flexner Report. Filling the team deficit in the short term depends upon *ad hoc* measures and altered sensibilities that will still remain long after better foundations have been laid in the formal medical education system.

David Lawrence suggests several categories of components critical to advancing team-based integrated delivery. Perhaps the greatest challenge, because it is the least mechanistic, is addressing the moral and ethical framework in which care is provided.[28] At the root of all successfully integrated delivery systems lies a subversive belief that physician independence and autonomy is in fact antithetical, even harmful to quality and safety. Because autonomy is considered unsafe, it is also believed to be unethical because it violates the Hippocratic oath and care result in deliberate or inadvertent harm. The notion that responsibility for the patient flows from sources of authority beyond any one doctor is not yet widely held in the profession. Moreover, it is something that needs to become equally plain among the lay population whose improved health is the purpose of the whole enterprise. Without agreement on this ethical foundation, without the willing ceding of autonomy, everything else dissolves into talk.

A second, more immediately thorny, challenge attends the need for systems of resource allocation and reward. The ways in which fee-for-service payment systems are blended with variations of incentive-based global capitation or incentives to the physician community (as at the Mayo Clinic) are labyrinthine. A third issue of greater political volatility yet is the need for whole series of decision-making and conflict-resolving systems that make it possible to take advantage of the tensions among various players whose unique perspectives are essential, without destroying the organization. The worst that can happen, when such systems are not in place and kept in good working order, is that organizations become stagnant or they splinter in favor of one powerful interest or another. Should this happen, integration disintegrates. Fourth, integration cannot happen without the technologies that enable real-time information sharing that can bring the evidence to bear immediately, and that render the entire care process transparent to patient as well as provider. Finally, there are "softer" but deep-running issues relating to public perceptions and patient education. Since Flexner at least, consumers have been socialized to think of a doctor—"their doctor"—as an independent practitioner and one whose competence was tied up in the fact of that independence, and to visualize "their care" as something centered in the doctor's office, where the doctor knows best and is clearly in charge. To think of health care in terms of "going to the doctor" at "the doctor's office" is a habit with a stranglehold. And so with quotidian perceptions of quality—that care is somehow less than the best unless delivered, one-to-one by the doctor—and not just any doctor, but *my* doctor. This suggests need for substantial educational, and marketing, efforts to change perceptions and persuade consumers into health plans with robust team settings and to stick with them for long enough to experience the superior results.

Devolution Ahead

All education rests on the ability and readiness to recognize distinctions, and so it does here. *Health care* as it offers itself to the twenty-first century—information intensive, institutionally complex, swamped by consumer expectations for transparency and participation, and in service to populations increasingly susceptible by chronic diseases—simply cannot be delivered according to the playbook written for *medical care* as it was offered to the twentieth century—acute-care focused, paternalistically delivered on the authority of promising but still limited science, and on the say-so of the men in the long white coats. The images from literature and popular culture, although quaint, are tenacious: the nostalgic company of Doctors Arrowsmith, Kildare, Welby, and all the remembered black bag-toting, house-calling pediatricians of our youth. They help fuel calls for the fashionable revival of the primary care and family medicine physician, nobly battling hegemony of the specialists who, although brilliant at the science of small things, come up short when it comes to the art of treating that elusive figure—"the whole patient." Yet for much of what is "primary care," an MD is not required at all, at least not up front, which is what makes such care "primary" to begin with.

A process of devolution is at work here. Once upon a time, and still in many places, the classically trained physician-scientist stood at the center of the office or the clinic—the mind to which all other minds deferred for judgment first, last, and always. Today, while this wonderful figure is not being banished entirely, there are unquestionably more centers of focus. This is because we know so much more science and how to apply it to medicine, and because patients, in whom patience once was a necessity if not a virtue, have become impatient health care consumers every bit as discerning and demanding of those shopping for cars or electronics. The effectiveness of teams, both in primary care and specialty settings, in which others besides doctors play large parts, illustrates this shift: It is the nurse practitioners to whom patients bond most closely at ASAP and who deliver most of the frontline care on a continuing basis. Nor would most cardiologists and cardiac surgeons, even those as highly-credentialed and accomplished even as the Churchwells, dare to presume today that they alone know everything necessary for the delivery of safe cardiac care.

Forces coalesce from several quarters to promote teams. In their still-developing role as laboratories for new models of care delivery, AHCs can lead by example toward team-based integrated care, both in their clinics and in their capacity as educators. As schools for the next generations of providers, AHCs cannot long escape the mandate to train providers in any other way. In 1910, science was the driver that promised to deliver medicine from empiricism and give it unprecedented therapeutic substance. The reformed medicals schools of the Flexner era were where this happened. A century later, science remains integral to health care, but translating it into useful service demands new models and new strategies. To practice in teams means to learn in teams from the start of medical school and throughout a career of continuous learning. Particularly for physicians, it means a different understanding of professional identity, one that encompasses familiar moral and ethical responsibilities, but with shared authority and, yes, diminished autonomy.

More immediate than educational reform, however, is this: Evidence accumulates that team-based care, particularly of those suffering from chronic diseases, produces measurably better outcomes than care provided by individual doctors practicing alone. That this is so even in the face of unfriendly reimbursement systems only amplifies its importance. Of course, science never ceases to look for cures. Meantime, the management of diseases for which there is no cure (yet) requires both more science and better organization. The product of this combination is what can be observed, for instance, in the improved outcomes for asthma patients treated in team-based integrated settings.

Both of these—the potential of AHCs as teachers of teams and integration, and the demonstration of superior clinical results delivered by teams already in action, at AHCs and elsewhere—are levers of change internal to the world of science and medicine as it merges into health care. An even greater force favoring teams and integration may be felt from outside medicine altogether. It originates in the business world, with private sector innovation, and promises to transcend many boundaries.[29] Wide-ranging innovations are already in effect, such as those affecting chronic disease management and large-population health care; innovations designed to push services directly into the hands of the consumer and to enable consumers to work with a variety of health professionals often in team settings. These kinds of changes are certainly disruptive, but they have a vast transformational potential for health care delivery across the board. The founding of new companies, and the involvement of large established firms new to the direct business of health care (Wal-Mart, Walgreens, CVS, GE, Google) accelerate delivery of integrated primary care to consumers using teams and technology. As this happens, the old equations operating as revenue, influence, and control, with regulatory and reimbursement regimes and questions of professional identity all come up for re-calculation.

Until now, remediation at the margins has trumped radical transformation, and progress has been piecemeal. "At Kaiser Permanente, we spend a fair amount of time re-acculturating physicians who come out of medical school and residency with little or no understanding of what it means to practice collaboratively, with physician colleagues let along with other members of the team," laments David Lawrence. "They are scientifically extraordinarily well-trained, but they really need to learn how to work with other people effectively."[30] And this comes from the good-as-it-gets environment that is Kaiser.

The science versus service dilemma addressed here sounds acute and contemporary. In fact, it is chronic and historical. It can be resolved, for the long future, only as past reforms won authority and, after a manner, permanence: through broad and deep institutionalization. How to speed that process for the closer future challenges today's AHCs as nothing since the Flexnerian reforms that created them and whose weighty legacy they still carry.

FOUR

Informatics Order

How to manage the enormously complex information environment of modern health care and still keep patients, who are the point of it all, at the center? How are physicians and other health care professionals to know, for every patient, how to do the right thing and just the right thing, every time just in time?

As the practice of medicine has come down to us over the past century in the United States, and as it has been taught in many places until very recently and in some places still is taught, the chief mechanism for knowing has been the individual human brain. The chief agent for applying knowledge to the diagnosis and treatment of disease has been the highly trained and credentialed medical expert, almost always a physician. The pattern, which became a model, was simple and deeply entrenched. From the first day of medical school onward, one read, one watched, one listened. And one ceaselessly "practiced," at first as an apprentice, eventually as a master. The process slowly yielded understanding, at the level that appeared at least to produce desirable and reliable (or reliable enough) clinical results. The model enjoyed a long, distinguished lineage. It was a longstanding quip among the model's skeptics that Sir William Osler was not the last medical man to think he knew everything there was to know. He was just the last man to have been right about it. And Osler died in 1919.[1]

Today in biomedicine, there is more to know than any human brain can possibly comprehend and act upon. The pace of accumulation of facts that shape clinical decisions accelerates to the point where the model of simply reading and then understanding has collapsed, even if it has not exactly disappeared. Sweeping up the rubble will take some time, for many practitioners still live amongst it, creatures of old habits and incentives not to change. But there is no other choice. By the late 1980s and early 1990s, a tidal wave of data-intensive biology had broken over health care, swamping clinicians with new and potentially useful knowledge. The amount of new knowledge that informs how a physician makes a diagnosis among the 8,000-plus known diseases, and then prescribes a medication or course of treatment, demands a radically different interface between science and health care.

In the absence of systems of clinical decision support, vast lists of data beyond the capacity of any one individual have left many a thoughtful and otherwise well-trained clinician with the problem of the unknown known. Every clinician can recount instances of egregious error committed because of something known but not known at the right time, something recorded somewhere but not accessible at the critical moment, something presented in such a way that it could not be brought within the scope of immediate decision making. Granting the presumption that the standard of care must always rise, ignorance has increased as information has multiplied exponentially. The fraction of knowledge that a person can comprehend remains constant, but the number of relevant facts per decision escalates. The more molecular the specialty, as with hematology and medical oncology for instance, the more intense the challenge.

System

In an era when innovation in medicine is synonymous with technology and health care takes on many of the characteristics of an information business, informatics—the science that deals with the structure, acquisition, and use of information—enables system.[2] A systems approach to health care rests on the family of informatics techniques, and when applied to both clinical data and the data of biological discovery, it smoothes the path from knowledge to utility.[3] While some physicians not trained in the culture of informatics resist it, finding it an affront to professional autonomy, many more find it empowering as it both takes account of their human limitations (chiefly, of memory) and takes advantage of the things that humans do better than the best computers (judgment and pattern recognition, to say nothing of compassion). Given an agile enough data-capturing infrastructure, it becomes possible, indeed routine, to verify desired outcomes through measurement, not just experience, of real world events that happen over and over again.

Informatics is instrumental and intensely results oriented. Like golf, which is not about the clubs but about the challenge of sinking a small ball into an obscure hole, informatics is not merely about recording things on computers but about the tough job of orchestrating an ever-changing evidence base toward the goal of improving standards of care and health outcomes. It enables practical systems of clinical decision support and pays back in improved quality, reduced variation, and lower costs. It represents a wholly different kind of club or set of clubs, to continue the golf analogy, and it has changed the game. At the time of Osler and Flexner, the union of science and medicine was still a halting affair, and even as it accelerated it advanced by what now appears random encounter. It was rather, observed one informatics authority, like NASA trying to put people on the moon by jotting down a rocket design on scraps of paper and then hoping that the next shift picked up the message.[4] A power shift has occurred, from reliance on the Post-It Notes of experience and memory to reliance on data—its capture, creative analysis, constant reuse, and refreshment.

Some institutions stepped up to the challenge more eagerly than others. One that was quick off the mark, Vanderbilt University Medical Center, in the early 1990s committed to what would become a large and lasting investment in informatics and the promise of restoring, for twenty-first century clinicians, the knowledge-mastery that Osler had claimed a century before. Informatics would interpret mastery differently however, relating to bodies of knowledge more transient than absolute. It was no longer possible (if in truth it ever had been) to know all things and a waste of resources to attempt to learn them. But with the right tools and technology, it was possible to master enough of the right things at the right time—and to know that everything changes and that change yields fresh information. Medicine is a practical art and science, physical and not metaphysical. The goal of those who practice it must be to know what one needs to know in any particular situation. This sounds modest but is not easy.

Vanderbilt was then in company of only a small band of academic medical centers and integrated health systems at the time, but has since set a standard. The ideas worked out there, and the lessons learned, model an information technology infrastructure with the power to enable the efficient diffusion of knowledge into the wider health care system at reduced costs.[5] In Flexner's time, such efficient diffusion had been easy to assume. Nowadays, it is not. Without such infrastructure, the health care system can only become even more dysfunctional. To know enough safely and effectively to practice old fashioned "just in case" medicine is no longer possible. Unless we master how to practice "just in time" medicine, cognitive overload will cripple and further disable delivery. To many critics, the present authors included, describing the American health care in the early twenty-first century as a "system" at all was a poor joke. Health care bedlam was more like it. "System" however at least has the merit of connoting reform when understood as "systems approach" to knowledge management and clinical decision-making.

Systems engineering is not new, and some of the best thinking about it in health care is borrowed from its application in other industries, notably aeronautics and defense. A systems approach offers similar advantages in health care to the degree that it holds potentially enables application of information to practice in a way that reliably improves individual clinical outcomes and the health status of individuals and of populations. In today's world, any health care enterprise that relies on autonomous individual practitioners and their reading and observations dooms itself to error and dramatically low rates of prevention, diagnosis, and treatment. In such context, the potential of systems thinking to do better is plausible.[6] In some cases already, the potential of systems thinking is well-proven. Like the systems approach to commercial aviation, where safety depends not on skilled aviators alone but also on embedded behaviors, processes, and tools that guide and support the individual competence of highly trained professionals and a low-accident occurrence rate. Further, a systems approach to health care can enable the clinical team and the patient, supported by the substructure of cooperation between basic science and clinical research, to achieve a comparable level of reliability and safety. Added up, such individual instances of top performance can improve the health status of all.[7]

The energy that in the old Osler model of autonomous learning and judgment was consumed by intensive individual education and patient-by-patient decision making, in a systems approach goes instead to guiding a network of evidence-based individualized care. Such system presumes a cycle. It begins with review of the evidence, which might be formal and graded (as in a research trial demonstrating one approach better than another) or experience-based (as in data based on the record of what was done in a number of cases together with clinical outcomes). The cycle next proceeds with design of a care process for what should be done, when, and how. Then, these decisions are rendered into electronic information tools suitable for use in the clinical setting. Process-control triggers and sentinel events embedded in the clinical workflow enable course correction in real time. Finally, all outcomes are banked and process performance is graded. Grading is key to continuous improvement and harvesting the insights of the changing evidence base.

The continuous improvement aspect of a systems approach to health care borrows heavily from techniques pioneered in the automobile industry first in Japan and exported globally beginning in the 1980s.[8] Medicine, once thought utterly recalcitrant to such discipline, proves not to be. In a systems regime, it is governed by one central rule: Quality (in aggregate, improved outcomes) must be built in to the care process at every stage, just as it was at every stage in the Japanese automobile manufacturing process. Never was quality something to be checked off an inspection list at the end of the assembly line. The information loop is endless, as information about subsequent service and performance history provides knowledge of real world outcomes that is folded back into the manufacturing process. Toyota's claim to make the best quality cars in the world was (until very recently) no mere assertion—they had data to prove it.

In an academic or other integrated health care setting, continuous improvement follows an analogous cycle to manufacturing, from data analysis and observation, to action, to display of clinical and process outcomes on electronic dashboards for use by all within the organization who have an impact on the final product. Accountability for each outcome is organic to the cycle, and the largest shortfalls between target and performance with the highest volume of cases—the weak links—become objects for evidence-based process redesign. Redesigned processes then feedback to a process dashboard to become real time controls on continuing performance.

A systems approach to health care requires the support of an executable knowledge base that encompasses the sum of current understanding and best practice. Knowledge in this form, to remain current, must in turn be supported by a cycle of evidence services. In the academic setting, this role falls to the library. The library is a largely digital one that provides search tools and a single source to published literature, guidelines, and databases. The library service is context-sensitive in the sense that it links the battery of information sources to clinical workflow so that relevant information can be supplied at just the right times, reducing the need to search. All search results are banked in the digital library for reuse.

The "Record" Challenge

The phrase "electronic medical record" achieved a level of public awareness in the early days of the Obama administration and, subsequently conjoined with the mandate for "meaningful use," became a procedural centerpiece of the Affordable Care Act of 2010. At first, it had stood apart from the broader campaign for comprehensive health care reform and was advanced as part of the economic stimulus package designed to combat economic retraction. The original measure called for spending $50 billion over five years to achieve the goal of electronic medical records for every American by 2014. In the tangle of what became the Affordable Care Act, this did not happen although the die was cast. The challenge was neither simple nor completely new.[9]

The first computer programs to store and retrieve patient records date to the late 1950s, and computer-based records were advanced as "essential technology for health care" by the National Academy of Science's Institute of Medicine in the early 1990s. Compared to other industries, medicine and health care have been extraordinarily laggard in their adoption and adaptation of information technology, with current surveys reporting that less than 20 percent of outpatient practices and less than 10 percent of hospitals employing even rudimentary computerized record systems at the end of the first decade of the new millennium.[10] And even these systems have not always had the desired effect, with reports of adverse clinical consequences due to the mismatch of particular tasks with system designs and implementation. At this still-tentative level of engagement and competence, the National Research Council was not optimistic about successful deployment of health care information technology adequate to the challenge twenty-first century health care reform.[11]

History holds other instances of the initially slow adoption of technology that, on the merits, would have seemed transparently virtuous. Forging a national, not just a regional, railway system in the nineteenth century depended on the easy connectivity of tracks belonging to different companies, which required adoption of a common track gauge. Alexander Graham Bell's invention of voice telephony could not become the "Bell System" without technical standards— what we hear with every dial tone—that made it possible for individual phones to "talk" to one another. And before the creation of key operating standards, the Internet remained arcane and limited to use largely by academe and the military.

Standards and connectivity issues similarly impede the electronic management of health information. Informatics pioneer William W. Stead, MD (director of informatics and professor biomedical informatics and medicine at Vanderbilt) and others set forth an approach to surmount this barrier to health information. Drawn from Vanderbilt's positive experience with electronic health records over the last decade, Stead's approach is also scalable beyond it.

First, it is important to understand the gap between expectations for electronic health records as enablers of a systems-based approach to health care, and the reality of most systems today. Then, it is critical to move beyond thinking of the electronic health record merely as a species of task automation to understanding it as a supple multi-dimensional tool for capturing data across biology, geography, and time. The result is a radically different approach with the flexibility to speed data integration, not just collection, and adapt technology to changes in people's roles and processes as they occur.

The Institute of Medicine's vision for twenty-first century health care embraced sweeping aims, calling for safety, effectiveness, patient-centeredness, timeliness, efficiency, and equity.[12] The vision contained several information-intensive challenges. As identified by the National Research Council, these range from comprehensive data on patients' conditions, treatments, and outcomes (the minimalist "historical" record); to cognitive support for health care workers and patients to help integrate patient-specific data; to cognitive support for professionals to help integrate evidence-based practice guidelines into practice; to integration of new instrumentation and biological knowledge into active learning systems that try new methods and apply patient experience as experimental data; to accounting for diversity among locales in the provision of care; to empowerment of patients and families in health care decisions, including custody of their own health records and direct and timely communication with professional care providers. Many of today's attempts at electronic health records fall short of even one or two of these goals, primarily because of the gap between the approach to their implementation and the variability and complexity of the clinical work experience.

The typical approach involves applying an off-the-shelf information system, which the health care provider to one degree or another then customizes, the goal of which is to automate care processes. The care process thus automated creates an electronic health record as a byproduct.[13] In this scheme, after-the-fact data entry is required if care happens to occur in some area of practice not yet automated, and the mapping of data into standard formats typically must recur practice-by-practice because exchange standards, while describing the identity of a data element (a drug orderable), typically fail to record what it means (ingredients, dose, strength). This approach can work, at least to a degree, in settings where both patient population and providers are self-contained. Even there however, in order to achieve quality and safety benefits of electronic records, providers must wait until the automation of each piece of the practice is complete and the record filled out. The very process grid created once automation is completed provides a barrier to change over time, as advances in science call for new approaches to diagnosis and as communities of patients and providers take new approaches to how they manage particular health problems.

In relatively well-understood and small enough-scale clinical processes where treatment regimens are clearly defined, such as hernia repair or cardiac angiography, the automation and transaction processing approach can play a useful role. Automation runs into problems, however, in more complex situations, where combinations of interdependent disorders demand more subtle problem solving and work processes. Here, different approaches are indicated. Proper connectivity can link people to one another and to systems. Decision support can make choices clear. Data mining can seek out relationships within data. Danger remains however of simply appending these approaches onto existing automation infrastructures. When this happens, the scale of knowledge and processes that can be accommodated inevitably shrinks. Mere automation of existing aspects of practice is not enough. Patient-centered health care calls for attentiveness to the intersection of multiple relationships across disparate bodies of information.

Medicine is a difficult challenge for information technology because, unlike physical systems, biological systems whether working well or poorly are highly variable, often changeable from moment to moment. As are the humans that embody these systems: No two people respond to disease or to treatment in exactly the same manner. Unlike in physical systems, in biological systems there are no strict laws that allow prediction of how behavior will recur in each and every set of conditions. Observation itself is fraught with variability and ambiguity. Without attention to the context in which events occur, the most careful observation can be wrong or incomplete. A blood pressure reading for example is far from an absolute value. It varies depending on the position when the measurement is taken (recumbent or standing), with the patient's levels of stress, and in the case of obese patients it must be taken with a larger cuff to avoid high false readings. In the pre-digital past, it mattered less that such contextual detail seldom appeared in paper records because, frequently, the doctor or nurse who created the record and treated the patient were likely the same person and already knew these things. Digitization of information and the advent of electronic records increase the chances that, as information moves around rapidly, such critical context will be lost. The danger extends beyond observation to laboratory tests, bioassays, and imaging results, where in the absence of context, correct interpretation of the data is difficult.

The constant addition to knowledge about biological systems and the diseases that beset them complicate the diagnostic challenge in particular. Clinicians interpret observations and weigh them against patterns in other patients in order to reach a diagnosis. New knowledge obviously requires new classifications, for which, if they are only subdivisions of old ones, the older, more aggregate record may still suffice. If they reference beyond prior classifications and demand new detail, however, then a different kind of record is necessary. Changing knowledge about diabetes is an example of how knowledge may migrate and make consequent records obsolete.[14] For purposes of tabulation, diagnosis codes, once upon a time, sorted patients according to common causes of mortality, or into groups as they related to the services required to support prospective reimbursement. If more detail was needed, a full, paper-based record supplied it. With the coming of electronic records of the sort focused on automation and by definition context-poor, the temptation persists to use diagnostic codes, in William Stead's warning, "*as if* they were [still] a more complete record despite the lack of clinical detail."

The complexity challenge accompanying the torrent of new biomedical knowledge rears itself up against a hardly-new backdrop: the chaotic, frenetic nature of clinical medicine itself. People, processes, and technology accomplish clinical work in the fluid context of changing patient populations and administrative demands. The contemporary clinic is a work environment that, if not utterly opaque, is far from transparent. Paper order sheets begin when a clinician orders care, diagnosis, and treatment upon admission to the hospital. Orders then change or are stopped sequentially, and before long it is impossible to access the sum of active orders in any one place. Consequently, orders are rewritten at major transition points, such as when a patient exits intensive care. While paper processes are typically the origin of electronic records automation, the transition is seldom seamless. As an example, a patient moves from intensive to intermediate care with a stop en route in the radiology department for an X-ray. Expecting that the imaging would have been done by the time of arrival in intermediate care, the clinician prematurely rewrites and cancels the imaging order. When the patient arrives in radiology, the technician finds no active order for imaging and passes the patient on without an X-ray. (With a paper record, the order sheet contained in the patient's chart would have physically accompanied the patient, and the lapse could not have occurred.) Of course, changing the program so as to prevent cancellation of imaging studies once a patient is en route to radiology could solve the problem—a "solution" however that reduces the flexibility that clinicians may later claim they need in a particular circumstance.

The cycle of problem identification and the addition of complexity to the system, which in turn presents a fresh problem, is not a fruitful one. Missing is realization of the potential of an electronic records to enable a new and simpler policy to begin with: In a case like this, as a patient changes levels of care, orders need not in fact be rewritten at all, but rather reviewed and updated with a single new entry confirming which service has occurred. Simplicity saves time, a precious commodity to everyone on the clinical team.

The fact that each member of a clinical team experiences the care process from a different angle reveals a further shortcoming of electronic records that are conceived merely to automate old tasks. Doctors and nurses pursue the same aims but, with different training and different responsibilities, they apply different uses to common terms. To physicians, the word *diagnosis* conjures first of all the cause of a patient's problem and thence the known means to cure a disease. Nurses contend first of all with a patient's experience as a result of disease and must reconcile their care of the patient, according to their own perspective, with the physician's diagnosis(es) and orders. Whereas the physician diagnoses, for instance, retinal detachment, which describes a cause, the nurse diagnoses visual impairment, a consequent disability to the patient's ability to function. Of course, visual impairment can have many causes and does not necessarily mean retinal detachment; moreover, a nurse may not diagnose visual impairment unless she actually perceives the patient to have a crippling sight problem. One diagnosis does not necessarily equate with the other.

Both language and clinical realities are subtle, and while clinical care follows, literally, a linear progression, along the way different actors play dif-

ferent roles and work with the script at different levels, adding their own details. Deciding on a course of action, the physician (or a nurse practitioner
or a physician assistant), for instance, prescribes a medication. Acting within the scope of that order, the pharmacist or the nurse dispenses the medication, determining how the course of action is to be carried out, thus adding
new details to the record. But if a change is required in the order, it must be
entered back at the originating point of the process, which with many electronic records regimes means that the detail of subsequent administration is
lost. A different kind of record is needed that dynamically connects such different perspectives and captures what will be inevitably changing contexts.

The electronic medical record must transcend mere information technology to become something than what the very word *record* can not convey. A
record implies a transcription of past events. As life experienced through time,
medicine is cumulative, and the "history" that a medical record contains, however intelligently automated, is necessary but not sufficient to meet the challenge of cognitive overload. To transform the idea of the electronic medical
record and its compass, it must be must be re-conceived as a personal health
knowledge base that is dynamic and oriented to the future rather than to the
past. Thus, a phrase like *field of knowledge* may be a better description than
record: a field without temporality and enriched by new information that is
folded in automatically when the knowledge of biology and health develops
in ways useful to the individual involved. The field of knowledge covers individual preferences, genetic make-up, best practices applicable to the individual, self-tracking, and, indeed, a "record" of care and outcomes. Such
a personal health knowledge base is both accessible to understanding by the
patient and to management by computer programs, and, when de-identified,
exports information to the world wide for global biological research. Without doubt, then, the principle of interoperability of health information is key.

The Interoperable Key

"Interoperable" and "interoperability" refer to a system of information management, unlike mere automation, that is capable of collecting and in-
terpreting both current and historical data and, as knowledge grows and

changes, a system that enables reinterpretation of that data. Such forward interpretation requires certain capabilities and that specific conditions be met.

First, there must be an accessible archive of raw material in various formats: voice, image, text, biometrics. Second, the data thus stored must be "liquid," that is, separable from home applications in order that they be useable by other applications. Third, data that are subject to one interpretation and one only and that do not change over time must be restricted to those interpretations. (Drug ingredients would be an example.) With these conditions met, it becomes possible to parse the electronic health record into its various components and thence to recombine and reintegrate them, dynamically and in real time, into frameworks that can serve multiple work purposes. Only when these conditions have been met will the cost and time required to implement electronic records decrease, while the flexibility to embrace changing roles, processes, and technologies increase.[15]

Where interoperability is at work on the ground day-to-day, computer algorithms and knowledge bases first detect clinically significant patterns in multi-source patient data. These are then presented to clinician and patient to make judgments about how to act, or not act, upon them. The computer interprets via computational techniques matched to the scale of the records capabilities and the clinical problem. When laid out in four quadrants, it can be seen how different computational techniques—automation, decision support, data mining and connectivity—scale and relate to records capabilities, and how different clinical activities draw from each of the computer's different techniques. Starting at the top with automation, for example, and proceeding clockwise around a circle through the other computational techniques, informed actions (as in evidence-based order sets and error checks) can be seen to draw upon both automation and decision support techniques. Pattern recognition (as for bio-surveillance) and visualization (as in disease management dashboards) draw upon decision support techniques data mining. Information access (the multi-source, multi-mode electronic health record in aggregate) draws upon data mining and connectivity. Distributed work (works lists and hand offs) draw upon connectivity and, to return to the top, automation.

People, in the end, still decide what is to be done. As clinicians become more familiar with the electronic health record, they will cease to see it as an automated tool but instead as a moving visualization of data through time, one that yields annotations to the record along with additional information tags. Everything, from the first data, to notes about context, to the latest tags recording a new fact, is archived in such a way that the now no longer merely historical record is left open to refreshment from the flow of discovery and newly observed patient data.

The use to which electronic health records can be put varies with the venue of operation, from health care entities that constitute integrated delivery systems, to regional health data exchanges, to personal health records and population databases. At the level of health care entities alone, where less than five percent of academic and community health centers in America use electronic health records in this way, the potential is enormous.[16] Still, only a handful of institutions have applied a system of computerized patient-specific clinical support: use by physicians particularly in the in-patient environment of an electronic medical records system backed up by event monitors searching for occurrences and patterns that humans might miss and to which they should be alerted. (Event monitors, combined with clinical decision support at the time of order entry when a physician is deciding how to act, either for diagnosis or for therapy, have been fully installed at Vanderbilt since 1994.)

The information architecture for the system visualizes a central communications management function (where, critically, data is "liquid" and separated from applications or tools) around which cluster and through which move component information resources. At the top sits the primary information resource of clinical workflow, itself fed by global knowledge. Other categories, from registration and eligibility to pharmacy and supply chain to revenue management, complete the system. Externally defined repositories of transaction databases and electronic charts are structured to make meanings explicit and accessible. Transaction processing systems are kept separate from workflow support and decision-support tools, which draw on many sources to enable displays specific to a particular situation. An example is the one-patient-at-a-time display. Viewed across the top, tabs permit drilling down into different categories of data, such as laboratory work or prescription history. A center frame presents new information about the patient in reverse chronological order and presents a disease management dashboard specific to the patient's problems. Across the bottom appear summaries of problems, medications, and allergies. Throughout, the data draw upon multiple systems both within and beyond the home institution.

Other patient-oriented display panels give access to groups of patients and enable different functionality in one logical operation. In the process-control dashboard designed for the ventilator management program, sets of colored flags describe the patient's status as compared to their health care plan, with green for a particular aspect of the plan that is within limits, yellow for a situation that needs action, and red for more troubling circumstances that could possibly spin out of control. Based as they are on data inputs from numerous systems, the flag indicators represent conditions in real time. And because such tools are insulated from automation components, they apply as called for across the care continuum whether inpatient, outpatient, or homebound.

Moreover, the principle of interoperability potentially makes the adoption of informatics-driven technology easier to begin. This is because it is no longer necessary for all clinical processes be automated all at once (or even at all). With this flexibility of initiation, it is possible to approach first those areas where work disruption promises to be the smallest and where resistance should be the least. Information technology is typically experienced as most helpful when it improves access to data, and is most resisted when it involves the dreaded task of data entry. The first stage at Vanderbilt therefore focused on straightforward information aggregation and data mining from a wide range of sources—images, scanned text, transcriptions, and text reports from data processing systems—for the purpose of creating a patient record. Filling out the resulting aggregate electronic health record took just four months and $500,000 to implement in 1996. First clinical use of this record can be equally non-disruptive. Clinical teams were presented with old-fashioned index cards with simple guidelines on the use of a web browser to access information as needed, if needed.

This first step is relatively easy because it leaves undisturbed the existing pattern of clinical work. Next steps, however, entail steeply rising learning curves punctuated by temporary dips in baseline performance at the point of implementation of each new stage. The dips represent the cost of learning to practice differently. While there was no dip with implementation of the records access stage (stage one), there is with subsequent stages: communication support, decision management and e-prescribing, and structured documentation. Team performance should never dip below the previous baseline, and rise successively with each subsequent plateau. This objective in practice raises the clinical team's expectations as improvement becomes visible. Health care entities will experience the stages of such technology change differently, depending on clinical priorities, prerequisite resources, and cultural characteristics. At the outpatient clinics, stage two (communication support) was implemented smoothly and resulted in substantial times savings for clinical teams operating in a large multi-specialty environment. Stage three (decision-management and e-prescribing) compensated for some cost in time with measurable improvement in quality.

However the sequencing of stages in different academic health centers and other integrated health care delivery systems may vary, their cumulative effect is similar: to build a pervasive digitally-enabled practice "ecology" and a culture of rising, systems-driven performance expectation. The same ecology is scalable beyond such local entities, a step that is essential to building an engineered health care delivery system that reaches beyond Flexner's paradigm of the natural transfer of knowledge into action, science into medicine, medicine into health. While the result is additive and in that sense linear, the process that leads there is, critically, iterative, open at every level to fresh data, new discovery, and constant contextualization. Examples exist of scaled-up successes, although they remain, in today's highly balkanized health care environment, still just examples.[17]

Build-Out

How interoperable systems of data capture and exchange can be related to participating health care entities at the point of care is illustrated by the MidSouth eHealth Alliance (MSeHA), in Tennessee. The framework can best be viewed through a series of stepped layers, starting at the bottom with infrastructure, which supports interventions in the middle, which lead to desired outcomes at the top. Infrastructure entails standards, which ease implementation of systems at the point of care by clarifying the meaning of data. As new data appears, it is tagged with standard terminology. Such data (record locators, medication histories, core laboratory results) then and only then can be shared, through data interchange, directly with participating point of care systems. As point of care systems absorb infrastructure-enabled information, new regimes of computer order entry, e-prescribing, closed-loop medication administration become possible and routinized. This supports, at the next step up, actual changes in practice, as care providers are empowered and incentivized to adopt systems approaches to care, to make evidence-based decisions, and strive for personalization of care. When this happens, the new level of value in health care as envisioned by the Institute of Medicine comes within reach: value that flows from safe, effective, patient-centered, timely, efficient, and equitable care.

That goal becomes less daunting, with the problem broken down into layers. The same simplifying approach can be applied to forms of governance as they relate to the progression from information infrastructure to medical interventions to health outcomes. At the foundation level of establishing and enforcing infrastructure standards, it is representative state, federal, and international jurisdictions/entities that must shape and govern process. The next levels, of data interchange and point of care where one population is targeted across institutional entities, alliances, and voluntary networks, are required. Higher up, point of care and change in practice fall to the realm of entities like practice groups and other discrete provider elements. At the peak, outcomes are managed and their value measured by payers and consumers.

The MSeHA employs its version of such frameworks, thus far at two levels of interoperability with the third to come, first to link the data interchange level with the point of care systems of participating entities. It does this through the concept of a network of information "vaults" within a common regional databank. Each participating entity (which could be a hospital or clinic, a group practice, a nursing home, retail pharmacy, or a payer) has a vault, containing records of transactions occurring in its respective local information system. These contents remain under its control. As information is updated in local systems, it passes through to that entity's vault in the regional databank. There it copies the content of those systems. Links are created within and across vaults to records with matching identifiers. An index updates in real time with the submission of new records and refinement of matching algorithms. In lieu of identifiers for each indexed person, which can add administrative management costs, a record locator service is used to search for similar records identifiable in the regional index. Upon deposit in a vault, each record is broken apart to permit concept-matching algorithms to tag clinical data by source and type, enabling tracking across different sources. It is important that participating entities at no point forfeit control of their own vaults, which keeps the system decentralized and flexible. On the other hand, it is also important that there be the opportunity for data mining across participating entities in order to increase the efficiency of a more centralized model.

The MSeHA approach also demonstrates how to achieve interoperability in stages. Stage two for instance extends into a regional integrated patient record of the individual patient's data available through a secure web browser, and cross-entity listing of patient encounters that were established in stage one. The key tool in stage two is disease management dashboards, and graphs of test results, across facilities. The extension function comes with the capability to show not only a result itself but also to reveal aggregated comparisons and variations from normal across entities and over time. MSeHA thus far encompasses such aggregated clinical data on more than 1 million patients from five hospital systems, two networks of community clinics, and one academic medical center professional practice group in metropolitan Memphis and southwest Tennessee. Emergency rooms, clinics, and hospitalists all have access. As soon as participating entities incorporate standards within their point of care systems, a third stage to achieve interoperability can be advanced, which will see data from the integrated regional patient records returned back into the point of care systems. Such back-and-forth movement of evolving data in real time—most broadly-based at stage one, then sorted into progressively narrower subsets in stages two and three—embeds interoperability into the frontlines of practice.

Themes of fluidity and flexibility that describe the development and operation of interoperable electronic health records within health care entities recur at the level of the personal health records tied to them. Digitization renders portable what once was stationary, or at least awkward and expensive to move around, and it enables individuals for the first time to collect and control access to complete pictures of their health status and the health care and life-style activities relating to it. This matters if health care is to evolve in less paternalistic and more patient-centered directions. The dual challenges of privacy and interoperability must be met, however. Personal health records and the electronic health records within health care entities must be linked and yet be kept separate.

One model to accomplish this begins with creation by an individual of a digitized personal record using an application service provider like Google Health. This begins with setting up a password-protected account and adherence to the privacy regime as stipulated by the service provider. The patient inputs multi-source, multi-mode information from experience and observation as well as from computer applications, sensors, even cameras. The resulting personal record relates to the electronic records of health care entities via the patient/consumer portals of each of the health care entities involved in the individual's care. With each of these the individual must also open and maintain a separate account. At this stage, the health care entities' privacy policies apply. Through portals, individuals can access parts of their records, communicate digitally with members of a clinical team, and obtain other services. Even as the portal supplies information, it also stands apart from the health care information systems that are its source. Thus, providers can respond to an individual's information submitted through a portal, but need not incorporate that information into the entity's internal electronic record.

Populations

Interoperable electronic records offer individuals—as patients, consumers, and citizens—the potential to participate more completely in managing their care while at the same time, granting providers access to the most timely and richest data with which to guide decisions throughout the clinical process. Such records change as information changes, whether it is information specific to the patient or information from ongoing biomedical discovery. These records enable the iterative refinement of clinical practice that is sensitive to context and that occurs in real time—that is, *in time* for medical interventions to make a difference to outcomes. At the individual patient level alone, interoperability in electronic records proves both a primary instrument and an enabler that makes the adoption of other tools easier.

Individuals aggregate into populations, and the research application of such information frameworks via population databases promises added benefits: pattern detection and recognition at the level of population scale and across a wide range of fields from epidemiology, phenotype-genotype correlations, and bio-surveillance to drug and device monitoring. At the individual level, information must be sufficiently specific to be particular and accurate. At the population level, however, the individuals who compose a population must in fact be de-individualized and the information in their electronic health record distilled out to form a synthetic derivative record useable for research purposes. Health Insurance Portability and Accountability Act (HIPAA) rules require removal of personal identifiers from records before they can be used for research possibly making it impossible to trace a synthetic record back to the original personal health record. At the same time, it must remain possible to continue to pass information forward from the active individual record to the synthetic one. This is accomplished with one-way hash algorithms, with the added safeguard of elements of disinformation to decrease further the likelihood of re-identification.[18] To meet the same caution, chronologies of events are preserved instead of actual dates of actual service, further masking identity. And in instances of diseases or attributes so unusual that they alone might trigger identification, these are purged entirely.

The logic of a population database framework can be represented schematically with two parallel columns of boxes. The one on the upper left represents all the information that would appear in an individual's electronic health record including diagnosis and procedure codes, test results, medication and notes. Directly beneath is a box indicating the step of de-identifying that record. Beneath that comes the box representing the result of de-identification, which is the synthetic derivative record. On the upper right is a box representing collection of biological specimens typically but not limited to blood. (At Vanderbilt, this occurs with every patient who does not opt out on the consent to treat form.) The next box down represents extraction of DNA from the tissue sample. And the third box represents the resulting DNA data bank. Interaction between the two columns of boxes comes only at this third level, between the synthetic derivative electronic record and the DNA data bank.

The same one-way hash algorithm is used both to tag the tissue sample and to create the corresponding de-identified synthetic record. This is what makes matching possible. Biological specimens from a small number of patients who do not opt out are excluded as disinformation, so that there is never precise knowledge about who is included in the data bank and who is not. For detecting causal relationships and associations, population-scale data are necessary, and such data and samples can supply them. On the other hand, for the targeted consented trials required to confirm causes or associations, identified data are still necessary. Because de-identified records cannot identify in reverse, in order to refer back to specific individuals in the electronic health record who might be benefit from discoveries or indicated changes in practice, it is necessary to back-search the electronic health record for all at-risk individuals whose profiles indicate notification and possible further clinical attention.

Penetration

If a systems approach to health care in the future is to come about, its information foundation must be laid with development of fully interoperable electronic health records. At every level, these must balance competing demands for compatibility and flexibility, much as the Internet saw explosive growth only following Tim Berners-Lee's invention of URL, HTTP, and HTML. All represented prescriptive standards although they prescribed as little as possible. They defined how information might be addressed, networked, and displayed, but they stipulated nothing at all about its content. It is such a system that must be replicated in health care, where standards—standards of practice, reference standards, terminology frameworks, and standard product identifiers, and vocabulary—assure a mutually intelligible digital language, and where metrics can assess end results as such interoperable information technology is put to use in real world settings.

It is unlikely that those settings will ever yield to quite the same level of interoperability of information that has been achieved in industries less dense than health care. In manufacturing and retail, it would be hard to overstate the power of the principles of interoperability—epitomized by the ubiquitous product barcode—to create efficiencies up and down complex supply chains and manage distribution and inventory with a precision and timeliness that makes what came before look crude by comparison. Brands may stay the same, but the organizations they represent need not necessarily supply the same products or services to all comers attracted to a brand. Movie rental business pioneer BlockBuster Video learned quickly that the value of its famous "torn-movie ticket" logo was only enhanced when it learned to track the tastes of its customers store-by-store and to customize its inventories accordingly. Convenience store leader 7-Eleven, whose very name communicated the long hours and ease of access that defined the essence of its brand worldwide, similarly learned that what customers want to buy in "convenient" settings varies and that local tastes and consumption habits dictated flexibility in inventory and pricing.

It is also difficult to overemphasize the urgent need to implement interoperability of information right in health care and to accelerate its penetration. Every business strives to tailor supply and demand. The more dense the industry context, the more challenging that effort becomes, and few industries are as dense as health care. The goal of interoperable health information and its application, beyond a few academic health centers and other already-integrated care providers and research institutions, make the feats of the retail world look elementary. The faster the knowledge base of science in medicine grows, the greater the risk that without interoperability the impact of discovery will be sub-optimized at best and perhaps even lost. Without success here, talk of "paradigm shifts" away from expert-based medicine to engineered systems-based health care will remain just talk. Tradition is tenacious, and the shadow of Osler and Flexner still reaches far in this regard, in the form of physicians and other care providers who have learned, from long training and experience, to function authoritatively and autonomously by remembering facts, assimilating data, and making judgments.

Tradition also attenuates, as is the case here. Its demise is probably inevitable as, practically, health care grows to rely on teams of people, processes, and information technology tools that function cooperatively to produce desired results consistently.[19] We have the tools, and we know the steps to take toward systems-based practice and care: targeting of high priority populations, gathering evidence into interoperable information systems, achieving consensus across institutions and among enterprises as to standards, definitions and metrics, measuring performance outcomes, and continually refining and refreshing the system as knowledge develops. It is an agenda that as clear and compelling today as it was when Flexner proposed, a century ago, the creation of a new-model medical/scientific expert. That model is now wanting and has become part of the problem. Yet, the way in which Flexner advanced his agenda remains as current as ever. To turn admonition into action requires examples so compelling that others will rush to emulate for fear of being left behind—or left out.

"The science is done," says Daniel Masys, of both informatics science in particular and biomedical science in general. The next challenge is "trying to change the world's practice."[20] "Done" may be a bit of an overstatement, but it is true that we have the knowledge and tools to manage science in order to make our knowledge count more quickly and more effectively in practice. We remain, still, much better producers of *new* knowledge, and then of early validation in clinical trials, than at changing practices in communities. This probably reflects the prejudice of American medicine since Flexner and of American health care at least since 1960s, a bias embedded in the private practice model where the individual physician/medical expert animates the system instead of the other way around. Where medicine is still regarded as the encounter between expert and patient, and where the relationship of that same pair may last for years, then continuity (such as it is) is thought of in those individual terms. As medicine strives to become genuinely patient-centered amid the information avalanche of genomics and proteomics, this arrangement will become untenable. It will be impossible for any one individual to know enough ever again to claim utter competence and to represent the apogee of care for which every patient hopes. Even the smartest people forget and make mistakes. Systems always remember and they reduce errors.

Lamenting the reluctance of the larger world for change, Masys reported a hospital where he had recently been admitted as a patient. He identified himself as working in biomedical informatics and was asked what that was. Another staff member piped in: "'Oh, I know. We have two broken EKG machines in your department for repair.' So that's the reality. That's where you send your bad infusion pumps. They still don't realize that they're working in a world of ideas and that the guidance that comes seemingly out of the walls really comes out of these systems that alert you when you're about to do something that we know is no longer the best practice."[21]

This is not to belittle what has already been accomplished at places like Vanderbilt. These facilities are the proving grounds for applying the principles of interoperability to the challenge of cognitive overload presented by genomics and proteomics. Their mission is to achieve better health outcomes. While these centers may still be relatively few number, the difficulty of what they have accomplished already amplifies the power of their example. They have proven, at some scale, that the principles of interoperability work and can make a difference. It is one thing to theorize about the scalability of innovation, to involve perhaps a few volunteers or a single clinic, and then summarize the results in a paper. It is the long leap to the next, middle level of integration that is critical. Large AHCs are one promising venue, places with thousands of employees utilizing systems and hundreds of physicians treating patients—large numbers of very knowledgeable people where prototypes of new ways of working square off daily with the unexpected and prove their worth. This is the hardest step, and it has been taken. Academic health centers have long since ceased to be the insulated ivory towers of Flexner's era. They are the "real world cement mixers" of health care, where interoperability has been shown to work.[22]

This accomplishment marks a threshold level of validity, perhaps not yet at the level of society, but one nonetheless fit for emulation. Proof of validity at the level of society does exist. Kaiser Permanente, the unusually large (for the United States) integrated care system that covers 8.6 million people, reports that digitization saves money and pleases patients.[23] And there is success in smaller admittedly more homogenous countries than the United States. The Nordics have had uniform electronic medical records systems approaches in place for more than a decade, which report basic outcomes data revealing the populations' illnesses, treatments, and changes in treatment protocols. Implementation across the trillion-dollar American health care field, with its intractable, "cottage industry" aspects of strong individualist bias and private practice tradition, is more daunting. Failure is more daunting still and will leave us like the man who willfully pokes himself in the eye and then complains he is blind.

FIVE

Ever Better

To heal the sick and to care for the healthy that they might stay healthy longer are the twin goals of medicine and health care. To reach them requires applying science to service in better ways. Product improvement and process improvement are ideas native to the world of manufacturing. They are most closely associated with enterprises from the industrial age whose purpose—pursued through sometimes simple, sometimes complex sequenced processes—was to produce physical goods. The term *goods* applies to such products because they represent higher economic value than the sum of the natural, human, and financial resources mustered to produce them. To create and sustain such value in competitive markets requires the relentless pursuit of improvement, or at least what can be marketed as improvement to consumers (something at which American car companies for years were notoriously expert).

Nothing, of course, says that the ideas of product and process improvement cannot be applied to the provision of services—such as medicine and health care—as well as the production of physical goods. The need is transparently great, for as many argue with good cause, the current delivery regime in America produces more "bads" than "goods": too many and too many poorly managed inputs turned into inadequate, uneven, unpredictable health output, something that the latest reform, the Affordable Care Act of 2010, has done little to change. That the way to improve output and the quality of the "goods" overall is to improve the processes of their production is now widely accepted at least in theory. It is best observed, in practice, inside those atypical organizations with scale enough to enable alignment of the supply of intellectual and financial resources, plus management expertise, with actual health care demand. Though as yet few, such settings shine a useful light on how to "make" medicine, and health with it, reliably better.

The examples that we illustrate below—and which are recommendations for teaching and learning at the AHC level, but are not restricted to it—follow no standard format. Indeed, each example evolved to a degree *ad hoc* in response to particular circumstances and fortuitous leadership. Even so, it is still possible to discern a pattern that is replicable.

In Cars

It is in connection with the prospect of process improvement that medicine's similarity, or dissimilarity, with other industries still stirs sharp debate. It is not just "old-timers" who demur that there is just too much that is subjective, personal, not "scientific" but "artistic" about what they do to make, for instance, the Toyota model of lean manufacturing seem even remotely relevant. Every practitioner knows that medicine is an inexact science, that every patient is different, that much medical practice is still frankly empirical. Reasons are not excuses, however, and a hefty literature now testifies to the appropriateness of importing to the industry of health care delivery processes of production proven to work making other sorts of things—like cars.

Automobiles have been described, famously, as the "the industry of industries,"[1] among the world's largest firms, and whose products offered a means of transportation that also allowed for unprecedented mobility and even self-expression. In its massive scale and the seemingly limitless appetite of its market, it resembled the energy industry to which its fortunes were closely linked. But it also resembled health care, which although not concentrated into a few dominant firms, was nonetheless large of scale and purveyed a complex product to a market of almost unlimited demand where consumers want quality and value. These two characteristics, one of the supply side and the other of the demand side, suggest strong transferability of techniques for getting the health care job done and for delivering goods better.

Twice in the twentieth century, the automobile industry led the manufacturing revolution.[2] In the years after World War I, mass production as practiced by Henry Ford at Ford Motors and Alfred Sloan at General Motors supplanted European dominance of what had been an artisan field and established America's twentieth-century economic predominance. A few years later, Eiji Toyoda and Taiichi Ohno of Toyota advanced the model of lean production, helping Japan recover from post–World War II devastation to become the second-largest economy in the world. At the time, each "revolution" came to be associated with its country of origin and attributed to certain national and cultural characteristics. These qualities proved largely mythical as it was demonstrated that there were, in fact, universal principles at work that thrived in native and non-native soils alike.

As the Japanese invented, refined, and inevitably exported it, lean production toppled both of the previous models of manufacturing. Mass production, in contrast to lean production, organized inputs of unskilled or semiskilled labor around the tending of specialized and expensive machines designed by a few skilled professionals. The resulting output was standardized products by the millions. Consumers benefited from lower costs of scale, but had limited choice. It wasn't quite as limited Henry Ford's famous "any color you want so long as it's black" dictum from the 1920s, but variety in mass produced automobiles during the American golden age of the 1950s and 1960s remained an oxymoron and was limited to cosmetics of color and yearly variation in tail fins and grill chrome. Because expensive, highly specialized machinery was economic only if kept running, mass production was a rigid system that demanded padding—extra workers, surplus of supplies, acres of floor space—to avoid disruption. Moreover, employees found the work deadening, hardly fulfilling except for its generous union-negotiated wage-and-benefits packages.

Before mass production, craft production dominated, turning out customized goods made by highly skilled laborers with relatively simple tools and using flexible methods and scheduling. The results were well-made, often exclusive, goods that consumers coveted, found aesthetically pleasing, and used for long periods. Quality was high, but so were costs, with the result that markets for the custom-made chair, for example, or the bespoke suit or the unique sports car remained relatively small markets for the elite.

Lean production was different. It drew on the advantages of both mass and craft production and re-combined them into something new and powerful. From mass production, it took low costs but discarded rigidity. From craft production, it took flexibility but avoided high costs. To do so required, above all, a different approach to labor or, as labor would be called in settings outside manufacturing like health care, "human resources" or "human capital." Its two predecessor models both had conceived of labor at the level of the individual worker. In mass production, the individual worker was relatively undifferentiated; in craft production, he was highly unique. However, in lean production, instead of seeing labor as inputs of individuals, whether as unspecialized or specialized, labor took the shape of teams with many different skills. Such teams, working with sophisticated, sometimes automated tools, produced as in mass production goods in great volume, and, as in craft production goods in great variety. It also produced goods of great quality and made mass customization possible.

And here was perhaps the greatest payoff of the lean revolution. In mass production, "good enough" (defined negatively as some acceptable level of defects across a narrow range of products) was deemed exactly that: good enough. Achieving higher quality than that, it was believed, would exceed the skills and motivations of "labor" and inevitably raise costs. In lean production, the opposite assumption held sway: Higher quality, meaning no defects whatsoever, tiny inventory, and a wide range of end products, in fact, drove costs down. "Perfection" early on became the much-touted goal of the lean production movement.

Skeptics saw this as utopian, even arrogant. Of course, nowhere has perfection been achieved in spite of being remorselessly pursued. It may be better to say that perfection lies in the pursuit itself and the process that facilitates that pursuit. Teams that level hierarchies, that call for learning ever-more professional skills, and that take greater responsibility for outcomes are the instruments of "perfection." This has proven so in the automobile industry, as it was remade in America, however unevenly from mass- to lean-specifications since the 1980s. It proves so, albeit selectively in health care—the "service of services" much as automobiles were the "industry of industries"—where since the 1990s borrowed understandings of process improvement have begun to be applied to the challenges of quality and costs.

Cars to Care

The language of manufacturing, whether mass or lean, is not naturally congenial to the world of medicine and health care. This is true at the most fundamental level and revealed in the question, addressed to most any doctor, "What is it that you do?" The replies—"To care," "to cure," "to serve," "to help," "to discover"—are the verbs most likely to animate a response. Not so "to make." It is no small irony that, like other professional services—law, engineering, accounting, architecture and, gradually, management—medicine and health care matured and indeed became "professions" concurrently with the very revolutions of industrial process that remade the material world in the nineteenth and twentieth centuries, even though they remained largely immune to the changes effected by these revolutions. Partly, this was a matter of scale: While some enterprises, notably steel, chemicals, and automobiles, adopted the corporate form early and became "big businesses," the professions typically went about their work in partnerships or even solo practice and remained, proudly, small. This was as true for the profession of medicine after Flexner's reforms as before them.

One consequence was a particular notion of service in medicine that has remained highly tenacious. It is axiomatic that no two patients are alike and that the relationship between doctor and patient reflects the unique individuality of both parties. There naturally arose a certain two-way possessiveness between doctor and patient. This is reflected in how people refer to this relationship. Americans in the second half of the twentieth century typically refer less to "the" doctor than to "my" doctor. Likewise, doctors have "their" patients. It does not oversimplify to say that medical care, thus understood, meant doctors looking after others for whom they had been given solemn responsibility much as a father, back in bad old paternalistic times, was responsible for his family (the difference being that patients unlike children could choose their parents). More a disposition than a model, such paternalism through the years delivered much fine medicine and great comfort to those in need. It was an attitude that did not, however, much incline practitioners to the notion that improvement might come about through some means other than by simply "being better doctors." It is suggestive that, through much of the last century, the phrase *medical progress* became embedded in the language of the medical profession (which saw itself at the primary agent of progress), while the word *improvement* did not. The former seemed easy to assume, as if in the natural order of things and conducive to "The March of Medical Progress...." The latter, which arose from the less lofty world of manufacturing, could not be assumed at all and seemed to imply some grubby effort to realize. To think about medicine as a process leading to improvement was something that few doctors had been formally taught and even fewer, from experience, had learned.

Virginia Mason Medical Center in Seattle is often held up today as an exemplar of process improvement in health care. Although not isolated, it is exceptional, beginning its trek to a new understanding of service with this critical admission in the words of CEO Gary Kaplan: "One of the biggest things that we learned is that we actually make things in health care. We make office visits and surgical procedures and laboratory studies and inpatient stays."[3] With that insight, it become possible to break work into pieces, to begin to understand how better to fit the pieces together, and so to improve the final product.

In reaching that point, Virginia Mason's history probably helped out. It was one of a small group of clinics dating to the late 1910s and early 1920s with roots in the group practice of medicine. Its founders came to the Pacific Northwest from the Mayo Clinic and the University of Virginia,[4] built their own hospital in Seattle and within a decade had established the first graduate medical education programs in the Pacific Northwest region. Today, it is a tertiary referral center for the vast swath of territory from Alaska to Washington, Oregon, Idaho, and Montana and is widely recognized for its culture of innovation and integration. It occupies a position as a sort of academic halfway house: Although not a university, many of its staff come directly from academia, including NIH, attracted to careers combining patient care, teaching, and research.

When Kaplan became CEO in 2000, one of his first projects was to orchestrate and conduct a board-driven strategic planning process designed to analyze several years of poor financial performance and to find a way to focus on the perceived need to treat the patient as a customer as much as a patient. At the time, this in itself was not unusual. The Institute of Medicine's reports wrestling with the issue of quality in care delivery, *To Err is Human* and *The Quality Chasm*, had been recently published and made for generally depressing reading. Virginia Mason, however, had long prided itself on attending to quality, or so it thought. Under Kaplan, the new strategic plan called for a pyramid structure that unambiguously put the patient at the top, while everyone else, doctors, nurses, technicians, took a subordinate position. In addition, it initiated a new physician compact that attempted to deal with misaligned expectations between what was necessary to progress and what physicians expected when they joined the group practice.[5] The compact was boldly admonitory and rich in the rhetoric of patient-centeredness, the need to "embrace change" and "take ownership" of a new vision of quality care and operating performance. But how actually to do it? Kaplan visited other medical centers and hospitals across the country, including the Mayo, Mass General, and Johns Hopkins, but was unsatisfied with all their management systems. A fortuitous meeting with an official from aircraft-maker Boeing, then still headquartered in Seattle, however, put Virginia Mason onto the tool that turned good words into the sustained process improvement needed to "make" better medicine.

This was the Toyota Production system, in use at Boeing and Wiremold, a wire harness company in Hartford and then one of the leading lean-manufacturing companies in the country. Kaplan soon discovered that what had been done there and at Boeing with "lean" had never really been attempted in health care. He decided to make Virginia Mason the pioneer. Senior executives, including all department chairmen and vice presidents, soon found themselves, in 2002, on the long flight to Tokyo to observe and absorb lean at the source.

Kaplan himself had never travelled to Japan before and testifies that the journey to Toyota City transformed his understanding in ways that the most intensive secondhand study back home could never do. To witness, on the Toyota floor-level, the manufacture of intricately complex yet "zero-defect" machines built for hard use, to see quality organically built into a process rather than inspected-for afterwards, raised for Kaplan countless likenesses to health care services as delivered, or as they might be delivered, at Virginia Mason. "I came home convinced that this was the management system that could take us to our vision to become the quality leader, which for us meant a zero-defect environment," Kaplan recalls.[6]

The Toyota production system "was totally obsessed with the customer," just as Virginia Mason claimed it wanted to be, in the name of quality and safety. What hit home the hardest was the way that the workers physically closest to the work were the ones improving it. Anyone on the assembly line had the power and responsibility to stop the process if something looked amiss. Staff satisfaction was high, end product quality unmatched in the automobile industry, and Toyota corporate financial performance the envy of North American companies—and not just car companies either.

At Virginia Mason, the Toyota production system was to become the model for a comprehensive management system, because in Kaplan's judgment health care lacked any other management approach capable of integrating multiple goals of putting patients as customers first, of quality, of safety, of staff satisfaction, and successful economic performance. In other words, this was not to be merely a project-based quality improvement exercise, but a system of thought and behavior designed permanently to infuse every part of the organization and every person in it with a zero-defect mentality and, according to the lessons of lean manufacturing, with the imperative to "make things" perfectly.[7]

"Seeking Perfection in Health Care" was the language Virginia Mason would use to describe this endless effort of institutionalizing quality.[8] To tour Virginia Mason's application of the Toyota production system to health care in its own setting is to be impressed not at its uniqueness but at its pervasiveness. Strategic leadership of course is important, but also inevitably transient. Long-term success in "achieving perfection" is less a matter of inspired quarterbacking than of endless blocking and tackling by everyone on the team. The team metaphor is deliberate, for although football is no Japanese obsession, the individual's submission to the group, i.e., the company, is central to the Toyota philosophy (and to Japanese business culture in general). Some critics have identified this as a debilitating cultural proclivity at odds with individualist cultures like America's, but this has proven not to be so. Taiichi Ohno's famous directive dictating the individual's behavior in a company—"If you don't have any wisdom to contribute, submit sweat; if nothing else, work hard and don't sleep. Or resign."[9]—is, in fact, not far from the credo of start-up and small firms that are the fertile seedbeds of entrepreneurship and innovation across many cultures. Toyota simply pioneered a system for applying the credo to large organizations.

As Toyota had gone about it, lean manufacturing promised daunting impact. It would halve just about every conceivable input and yet improve the value of output, measured in lower costs and higher quality: half the human effort, half the space, half the equipment, half the inventory, half the investment, half the engineering time, and half the new product development time. The enemy throughout was waste, or just the "padding" that the business world had gotten used to in large, inflexible mass production systems. Vanquishing waste required seeing it in all its different manifestations.

Ohno had counted a circle of seven vulnerable points at Toyota: overproduction, time on hand (waiting), transportation, processing, stock on hand (inventory), movement, and defective products. Virginia Mason translated each of these concepts to the health care setting. Lab tests were a clear instance of wasteful overproduction, patient transfers of wasteful transportation. Charge tickets were a clear instance of overprocessing. Drugs and supplies typically led to bloated inventory. Looking for paper charts was a clear waste of motion. Too many large and centralized machines looked like wasted engineering, while professional liability was the simple consequence of the waste of making defective, poor quality products—or of delivering defective, poor quality services to begin with. Making the logical connections at every point between manufacturing cars or airplanes or air conditioners and delivering health care involved only a modest imaginative stretch. For what was modern, science-intensive health care if not an elaborate combination of complex production processes, ranging from admitting a patient to conducting a clinic visit, going to surgery, or sending out a bill? Each of such "products" involved numerous discrete processes, many of them very complex. And all of them requiring concepts of quality, safety, customer and staff satisfaction, and cost effectiveness. Should any one of these fail, the result could be an error leading to avoidable patient fatality.

Virginia Mason in time embedded these connections into its own "production system." Although it grated at first on some traditionalist ears, use of the word *production* was a critical and deliberate choice. Virginia Mason defined its product as impact on health outcomes. This was something no less tangible and no less measurable than the turning out of a new cars. This production system was designed to flow simultaneously through several channels.

"Value Stream Improvement" looked at the linear flow, in space and time, of regularly repeated events. In the emergency department, for example, Value Stream Improvement considered patient movement from ambulance to bed-assignment across what were originally at Virginia Mason eight steps, probing for wasted effort, poor communication, and weak hand-off points. The resulting Value Stream Map called for reducing eight steps to six. Value Stream ideas for improving nursing efficiency included input from working nurses, who addressed everyday problems such how to handle the disposition and logistics of patient handling in hallways and nursing stations. An idea emerged for nursing "cells," or rooms of close proximity enabling nurses and patients to relate in a more synchronized flow. The result was better patient surveillance, fewer call lights, and a leveling of the load across cells which was especially beneficial for handling high-risk patients. As process improvement, nursing cells yielded highly quantifiable results measured, literally, in steps taken and saved each day. Over three months, nurses reduced their "travel" from 5,818 steps to 846. Patients reduced theirs by half, from 2,664 to 1,256, and the patient dissatisfaction rate fell from 21 percent to zero. Both nurses and patients spent radically less time in indirect care (nurses' time falling from 68 percent to 10 percent; patients' time from 30 percent to 16 percent). The time RNs spent gathering supplies was cut nearly in half, from 20 minutes to 11. In total, RN time available for actual patient care reached an all-time high of 90 percent.

"Rapid Process Improvement" systematized the search for changes that could be made quickly and entailed continuous team workshops that included disciplined week-long exercises using lean techniques to achieve immediate results in the elimination of waste. From consideration of Ambulatory Specialty Scheduling to Skilled Nursing Placements to Inpatient Medication Integration to Rehab Medicine Patient Flow, the target areas for Rapid Process Improvement were nearly endless. One useful mnemonic, "5-S" meaning sort, simplify, standardize, sweep, and self-discipline, addressed workspace organization, or typically disorganization. At Virginia Mason, the test case illustration was the anesthesia "shadow board" before and after a 5-S makeover. *Before*, we see a prep surface perhaps best described as one of randomly mixed items, some of them draped and thus not quickly visible. 5-S asked workers to separate what was necessary from what was not (sorting), then to create a fixed place for everything that remained (simplifying), then to control the work area visually and physically (sweeping), and finally to document procedures and agreements made during previous steps (standardizing). The result was self-discipline, the fifth "S," and sustained, structured follow-through on all 5-S agreements.[10] *After*, we see a very different prep surface of clearly labeled and segregated instruments and supplies, where it would be impossible to mistake one thing for something else.

"Standard Work" focused on the operation of any individual worker or, in lean language, the single team member. The idea here was to ensure that work and work expectations were both safe and reasonable by learning to detect undesirable conditions as soon as they occurred. Future improvement efforts, and easier staff training, could be built only on this foundation. The standard work analysis cycle adapted from Toyota first was to observe and understand the work and record its time and other requirements. Then, it was possible to analyze the work and identify waste. Then, it was possible to eliminate the waste. Finally, it was possible to standardize a new repeatable work cycle free from waste. Using central line insertion as an illustration, the Virginia Mason Production System depicted before, during, and after steps. *Be-*

fore meant a work surface clearly organized and labeled to 5-S standards, and dry prep of 30-second hand scrub and 30-second dry, or a 2-minute wet scrub and a 1-minute dry. *During* depicted universal techniques for maximum barrier protection including drapes and gloves, followed by application of either transducer or manometer methods of insertion. *After* called for dated and initialed "Approved to Use" indicator and completed paperwork sorted in yellow color to the top of the patient chart, and in white to the chart's progress notes.

To see must also be to do. In order to make a difference, the ability and proclivity actively to seek out and identify subpar components of complex processes, which the "Standard Work" principle embodied, presumed the ability to take action. At Toyota and similar manufacturers, "stopping the line" defined this responsibility: The understanding that any worker at any point along the moving production line could halt the entire line in order to correct a mistake before it became hidden in the finished product or before units behind it became subject to the same error. "Stopping the Line" became at Virginia Mason the "Patient Safety Alert System," in which any worker—not doctors alone—could stop the process. Increasingly, many did, with safety alerts distributed widely across functions from the highest number (in 2008) having to do with systems (38 percent), and the lowest to do with equipment and facilities (3 percent). In between, alert workers flagged safety problems related to diagnosis and treatment, often concerning medication errors, as well as matters of security and personal conduct. From the first implementation of the Patient Safety Alert System in 2002, alerts rose from 3 per month to 237 per month in 2008. This suggests the value of vigilance, and how the involvement of the people who perform the work can radically transform procedures and systems once deemed acceptable and safe.

A presentation made to introduce Toyota's production system to health care at Virginia Mason gave several examples of the "raw material" fundamental to process improvement. Under the heading "Key Concepts: Understand Value," appears a much scrawled-upon chart titled "Value Stream Map for Surgical Case Cart Preparation." It is a photocopy of a working paper, revealing in its very incompleteness the truth that process improvement is an endless work-in-progress. Abbreviations—CT, LT, PT, CO,VA, NVA (cycle time, lead time, processing time, change over, value added, non-value added)—pepper this paper, matched with the figures determined for, in this case, cycle times and value added for each of eight steps in the prep process: Obtain case cart pick list;

prepare case carts; pick sterile supplies; transfer to cart; pick instruments; sign list cover label cart; gather missing instruments; stage carts for delivery. Most striking, however, the study team has crossed-out three of the original eight steps (prepare case carts; transfer to cart; and gather missing instruments) and calculated the time saved and waste reduced: "10:34" down to "6:12." Each of the three steps edited out had produced zero percent value added.[11] Each of the five remaining steps was calculated to produce 50 to 100 percent value added. And yet, there it all had stood: that which was the most valuable yoked to that which was the least, until careful deconstruction and measurement revealed the obvious.

Most obvious of everything that was learned from Virginia Mason's appropriation of the Toyota production system was the interconnectedness of goals. Delivering quality, safe, and efficient care was one process. Virginia Mason today consistently places in the Leapfrog rankings of top urban hospitals.[12] That list is notable for its recent requirement that top institutions demonstrate leadership in both quality and efficiency. The Toyota production system and lean manufacturing discovered this long ago: Efficiency without quality, and vice versa, was simply impossible. Each led ineluctably to the other until the two terms and the ideas behind them merged into one. Thus, quality of care rose not just concurrently with but also intermeshed with the operating margins necessary to secure the financial future of the institution and sustain yet more process improvement. In 2000, before starting down the lean manufacturing path, Virginia Mason's margin was nil. In 2006, it had risen to 15 percent, by 2007 to 20 percent. The numbers—both of dollars and of the infection rates, the two benchmark safety practices of clinical quality—betokened a shift in management thinking that still seems radical in American health care. It was, and is, radical because it is deep. "Management" had ceased to be the exclusive province of administrators but devolved outward and downward through a more responsible organization: "stopping the line" has, it turns out, management-level consequences. Where managers once controlled, they now taught and engaged the other staff who did the quotidian, value-added work. Organization fixation on the departmental work unit gave way to value stream optimization. Shallow process knowledge became deep process knowledge. Quality problems became quality commitment. Localized, tribal knowledge became standard work and training guidelines. The instinct to add staff in order to solve a problem changed to a deliberate attempt to eliminate waste first. Confusing or minimal feedback became fluid information flows across every workspace and process. Impulsive triage and firefighting fell away before methodical fire-prevention. The assumption that the provider necessarily knew best what a patient wanted gave way before active patient involvement.[13]

For Kaplan, the impact of Virginia Mason's production system was nothing less than "changing the mind of medicine."[14] What's more, in 2008, Virginia Mason established an educational institute for training others from around the country and the world in its lean production system.[15] For many providers, lean manufacturing remains a possibly elusive future goal, but its fundamental directness gives it the realistic potential for realization. The Toyota Production System did after all "change the mind" of manufacturing, consigning mass-production skeptics to obsolescence and decline. With the proven transferability of such process improvement to health care, minds should change. The new participatory, transparent, open-architecture reality of organizations like Virginia Mason looks nothing like medicine's old citadel and indeed rebukes it. (A. J. Cronin's 1937 novel *The Citadel*, set in early twentieth-century England, ends with depiction a particularly heinous and fatal error as a patient dies needlessly on the table: fictional truth-telling at its most powerful.)[16] Patients not providers come first. Evidence-based, defect-free care banishes errors once tolerated as collateral damage. Real-time, stop-the-line quality assurance replaces end-of-the-line inspection and repair of errors already made. Time, once thought abundant and thus used often wastefully, becomes the most priceless commodity of all.

A Japanese advisor once visiting Virginia Mason was baffled when he encountered the patient waiting room. "What is it for?" he asked. On being told by his American host that all hospital departments had them, he shot back: "Aren't you ashamed?"[17] Waiting for an appointment, waiting for test results, waiting for a bed, mostly just waiting for the doctor in the waiting room are clichés of the culture of medicine and health care as it evolved in the twentieth century. This is true largely irrespective of payment regimes, from Britain's single-payer National Health Service to America's scattershot, elaborately subsidized "private" insurance-based system. The Japanese trainer's question rose not from any particular sensitivity to the inconvenience that waiting causes to the patient (though it surely is such), but rather from the inefficiency that waiting signals in the system. It is the red flag that the wrong system is operating and that value is being eroded not enhanced. "Perfection," as promised in the creed of the Toyota production system and its Virginia Mason manifestation, may yet be a way off in health care, but it need not be a chimera. At places like Virginia Mason, there are strong enough intimations of perfection. "We have," Kaplan reported proudly in 2009, "just built a new ambulatory clinic with no waiting room at all."[18]

Hybrid

Virginia Mason is an example of how a single methodology of process improvement, the Toyota Production System and the doctrine of lean manufacturing, can deliver care more efficiently, improve quality and lower costs. It is a single, highly concentrated instance of how to enable the delivery system to improve value: the quality of results relative to the cost of inputs required to achieve them. Efficiency in the application of natural, human, and financial resources for production of goods and services must be the goal of every business that aims to stay in business. In market economies, even highly regulated and imperfect ones like health care, what is gained today can be lost tomorrow (and frequently is), and the quest for value must be persistent and unending. The lean mantra—half the human effort, half the space, half the equipment, half the inventory, half the investment, half the engineering—begins to convey the radicalism needed to increase and sustain value or, perhaps simply, to rescue it.

Hybrid approaches invite consideration, too. The Geisinger Health System (GHS) in northeastern Pennsylvania affords insight into combinations of processes, in its language of "improvement methodologies," to tackle the value challenge. Again, setting and history are important, and GHS admits to some fortuitous institutional circumstances that have enabled it to set forth exceptionally robust efforts at process improvement. Founded in 1915 by the widow of iron magnate George Geisinger and designed to emulate the Mayo Clinic, GHS is an integrated delivery system that employs more than 20,000 people including a 1,000-member multi-specialty group practice at seven hospitals and two research centers and numerous practice sites across northeastern Pennsylvania. The system also includes acute-care hospitals and specialty hospitals, ambulatory surgery centers, and abundant outreach services spanning prenatal care to the needs of the elderly.[19] It also has its own 448,000-member insurance company, the Geisinger Health Plan. Unlike Kaiser, GHS is integrated but open, its services available to non-Geisinger Health Plan patients in its service area, who through other payers, public and private, represent a majority of GHS's patient-care revenue. Less than half of the health plan's members are actually served by GHS physicians, the rest are under the care of a broad network of non-Geisinger physicians and other regional hospitals. Likewise, just one of Geisinger's three acute-care hospitals is closed-staff. This integrated yet open quality, the fact that Geisinger embraced both a delivery system and an insurance regime, and its location in a region where the population is statistically older and sicker than national averages, encourages alertness to market opportunities and a proclivity toward innovation.[20]

Cancer surgeon Glenn J. Steele, president of GHS since 2001, formerly vice president for medical affairs at the Pritzker School of Medicine at the University of Chicago, brought to the job firsthand experience with patients, access to care, challenges to physicians of providing timely and adequate care, the peculiar needs of education and research, and the shifting reimbursement landscape. He came to rural Pennsylvania attracted by GHS's integrated delivery and insurance system and the opportunity it presented to experiment, in a contained and controlled setting, with processes to increase efficiency of care delivery, raise quality, and so ameliorate value. Of course, the vast bulk of American health care delivery is emphatically not integrated. Even so, AHCs are more integrated than most of the industry and so are doubly obliged to look closely at how GHS has force-fed process improvement in the pursuit of improved value.

In testimony to the US Senate Committee on Finance in 2009, as debate on health care reform was just beginning under a new administration, Steele made policymakers aware of the immensity of the structural challenges to higher-value care delivery. Care was hugely variable and highly fragmented across localities. Information transfer, the hand-offs that occur when patients move from one part of the system to another, was disjointed with large cracks for all but the most agile and well-informed to fall through. The payment system rewards units of work performed and numbers of patients seen but ignores patient outcomes.[21] He offered examples of how GHS re-designs care delivery through process innovation and the principles that can be extracted from the experience. Probably the most visible example, if only because headlined in the *New York Times* two years before, illustrated how in the American delivery system it is normal for providers to get paid, and get paid more, for making avoidable mistakes.[22] "This does not happen in other businesses," Steele bluntly told the senators. "Why are health-care services an exception?"[23]

To reach the problem of perverse payment incentives and demonstrate the potential of effective care re-design, GHS examined the processes for delivery of elective cardiac surgical care, specifically coronary artery bypass grafts (CABG).[24] There were three steps to "making" the product, each documented in the professional literature as reform proceeded. As would be done in lean manufacturing, the analysis began by breaking down the component tasks needed to "make" a complex product (a heart bypass) and discovering areas of waste. In practice, this meant turning guidelines into actions, the performance of which could be implemented and checked. The guidelines drew on a combination from the American Heart Association and the American College of Cardiology, and from them GHS distilled forty steps supported by the evidence-base that would define this procedure for each and every patient undergoing it. All forty steps were then incorporated into GHS's electronic health record system, which took on a watchdog function, signaling the omission of any identified step or, if the clinician proved, documenting the reason for making an exception. Transforming the guidelines into a checklist demanded multiple inputs from across the organization, which brought into play not only diversity of advice but also the multidisciplinary teams to implement it. A clinical leadership team took responsibility for developing the specific care process steps that were to be followed. A clinical operations team tackled the insertion of those steps into workflow process and flow sheets, with team members representing various functional areas: clinical, operations, information technology, and process improvement. Concurrently, a steering committee team conducted financial analyses, established pricing, and monitored claims and administration. This was step two: establishing a risk-calculated, essentially package price for a defined medical/surgical outcome, rather than a piece-rate price for a certain set of procedures. The conceptual difference between this and the old DRG (diagnosis related group)-type pricing is hard to overstate. The new method of pricing covered the whole continuum of care that the evidence-based guidelines, or GHS consensus of best practices, experts said would yield the desired outcome for most patients all the time. In addition, it guaranteed that providers would act uniformly at all times in accordance with the guidelines.

The package started with the initial visit with the physician/specialist, extended through three months of post-operative care, including cardiac rehabilitation, and covered all hospital costs for the surgery in between. There was no fine print. GHS assumed all the financial risk associated with complications and any need for re-admission. Failure to perform entailed serious financial consequences. Indeed, re-admission became a tacit confession of the provider's failure to meet its part of the care understanding. This understanding was part three, represented in a formal compact signed by GHS and the patient or the patient's family, enjoining patient education and generally underscoring the partnership between patient and provider.

GHS dubbed the program "ProvenCare," connoting its foundation built on evidence-based, best practices and communicating its ability to deliver what is promised. This was not without some awkward discoveries along the way. While GHS's performance was already above national averages for cardiac surgery outcomes, it still turned out that 40 percent of patients did not in fact receive all 40 best-practice steps. Not even GHS, it seemed, was as good as they thought they were—until they broke down the process and discovered what pieces were missing and where. Ultimately, however, the discipline worked and within months the performance number hit 100 percent and stayed there. From this fact, all the right figures then followed: Complications dropped 21 percent, infections 25 percent, re-admissions 44 percent. With better outcomes (higher quality) achieved for less effort (fewer inputs, or inputs more efficiently arranged and dispensed), costs fell and hospital stays were reduced by half a day.[25]

"ProvenCare" and the idea of warranting acute-care medical and surgical performance- based on outcomes has thus far been applied only within the fully integrated Geisinger-insurance population, but it has been expanded there beyond heart surgery to other acute-care areas, including heart catheterization, hip replacement, obesity surgery, cataract surgery, prenatal care from conception to birth for babies and mothers, and evidence-based use of high-cost biologicals such as erythropoietin. In each instance, the same pattern has been observed. The better the research into how to deliver care and the better the EHR-enabled discipline in adhering to the prescribed practice steps, the higher the resulting quality and the lower the costs.[26]

American health care generally excels at acute episodic care, and Geisinger's innovations demonstrate the added potential of expertise when embedded in process. With chronic disease, for which the American health care delivery system is considerably less adept, Geisinger demonstrates how the same combination of evidence-based, best-practice thinking with disciplined process improvement can optimize outcomes. In the case of high-prevalence chronic maladies—diabetes, coronary artery disease, congestive heart failure, kidney disease—the aim is less to cure than to limit disease progression, something undergirded at Geisinger by a programmatic focus on preventive care. Much quotidian chronic care calls for nurses and the Geisinger initiative centers to standardize care protocols via electronic tools that enable, for instance, nurses to capture and process clinical information before patients even enter the examination room. "Eliminate, automate, delegate," themes embedded deep in the culture, drive every preventive program. Geisinger's EHR literally enables them, incorporating patient care plan needs directly into doctors' order sets. The EHR also has a maintenance alert function and aggregates to a single screen "snapshot reports" of specific conditions in real time.

Streamlined and measurable, preventive care is the result, and "bundled" care the instrument that achieves it. Success is defined only by the compliance with all performance metrics in the bundle. Nine evidence-based care requirements are required for diabetes patients: glycosylated hemoglobin (HbAlc), low-density lipoprotein (LDL), blood pressure targets, smoking status, urine protein analysis, influenza, and pneumococcal vaccinations. Before they ever cross the clinic threshold, diabetic patients and their respective circumstances have been identified electronically. One click of the mouse enables the physician to verify and accept evidence-based order entry sets for each individual patient, which include standing orders for routine tests (such as HbAlc and LDL). The system provides automated reminders to both the clinical team and the patient, along with an option for patients to self-schedule appointments, to review post-appointment summaries, and set of self-tracking goals with positive and negative feedback. With Geisinger's multiple clinic sites, it is a critical feature of bundling that performance reports are distributed electronically to all practice sites. Moreover, these reports compare, for all to see, the performance, against historical trend and peer sites both of a practice-sites *and* the individual physician. In 2006, Geisinger began to track its performance in meeting 100 percent of the bundle of best-care requirements for diabetes patients, while at the same time, primary caregivers opted to link their compensation to the number of times that their 25,000 diabetes patients receive the full bundle of care. Results were two-fold and synchronously virtuous. Statistically significant improvement could be observed in patients receiving the optimal levels in the practice bundle for glucose control, blood pressure, and vaccination rates, trends that for the long term are promising. Providers for their part, having agreed to sever the link between their pay and the number of patients seen each day and the number of procedures done and tests ordered, looked to new incentives—up to 20 percent of cash compensation per physician—tied to patient satisfaction and quality goals as objectively expressed in improvements in bundle-scores. Geisinger's process-driven efforts to optimize chronic disease care can also be seen in its approach to chronic kidney disease and the associated problem of anemia, where through remote-care management and application of a pharmacy-based model achievement of desirable hemoglobin ranges increased, and the numbers of units and the cost of the erythropoietin needed to control it fell.

Waste destroys value, which must increase if better outcomes are to be achieved. Process improvement makes value creation possible, but only if it is conceived as continuous re-design. The "solution" that works best today may not, given new evidence, work best tomorrow. Therefore, Geisinger's concentration on what it calls an "innovation infrastructure" enables development of new care models even as it assumes that these models will be replaced by newer ones as evidence changes and technology improves. Just as obstacles to transportation infrastructure—highways, railroads, air-traffic control—impede movement and prevent interconnectedness, so these same obstacles hinder commerce. Process infrastructure, too, drawing from the Geisinger experience, must meet minimal, yet ambitious, structural standards if it is the carry the load of change and innovation needed to deliver better service and higher value. This infrastructure must rest on the foundation of an integrated delivery system of facilities, health plans, and physicians capable of multi-specialty collaboration. It must possess entrepreneurial clinical leadership that is unafraid to experiment (and sometimes stumble) and that is engaged through linked non-fee-for-service-based financial and nonfinancial incentives. And it must embrace nonproprietary and interoperable electronic health records systems essential to centralized continuous innovation, decision, and quality support and patient empowerment. In this particular, integrated delivery systems such as that of Geisinger must lead the way for the many small practices and independent hospitals that still make up most of the nation's health care delivery capacity.

Variations

Abundant resources exist to do this now, perhaps the most renowned being Donald Berwick's Institute for Health Care Improvement (IHI).[27] Much has been accomplished since the foundation of IHI in the late 1980s, when the notions of quality improvement and industrial process were utterly foreign to most US health care settings and were greeted with hostility by much of the medical profession. Indeed, today, the opposite view prevails, but when IHI was just getting started in 1991, Paul Batalden co-founder and quality pioneer at Hospital Corporation of America, predicted it would take at least twenty-five years to achieve broad impact.[28] This proved correct in a manner of speaking, for the feeling lingers that by the point at which estimable organizations like IHI can engage the problem, those organizations are already playing catch-up. The rancorous debates over health care reform in 2009 and the Affordable Care Act that resulted could not have made it clearer that we are still not where we want to be, or even anywhere close. The "system" still isn't one, and too many of its component parts threaten to keep it dysfunctional. The promise of leadership offered by providers such as Virginia Mason and Geisinger depends on the presence of willing followers.

Critical as it is to better outcomes and broader impact, process improvement teaches above all that transformative change begins at the beginning. It means starting again. It does not mean repair work: that is, inspecting for and then correcting embedded errors. At Virginia Mason, the Toyota system did not fix problems as such—it remade an institution. At Vanderbilt, an even older institution, starting again would demonstrate how re-purposing an organization around system-wide, continuous improvement goals and finding the right tools to measure its progress, required evidence-based leadership as well as evidence-based medicine in order to make the impact sustainable and permanent. The leadership looked outside for help and found it in The Studer Group, a Florida health-care consultancy with clients such as the Cleveland Clinic. Founder Quint Studer was a teacher-turned-health-care administrator who had come up through hospital administration ranks, absorbing the idea of improvement as a way of life and work. His pragmatic program aimed to do three things: improve employee job satisfaction, improve the quality of service rendered to patients, and improve the financial performance of the organization. Money, though important, was not the center of the Studer scheme, but a consequence. (At Vanderbilt, it would have been disingenuous to deny the importance of money which financed research and supported the business model sustained by its clinical enterprise.) Across Studer's varied client base, the process had the effect of realigning what he saw as the fundamental idealism of health care with the reality of how hospitals and medical centers actually could be motivated to practice and deliver it.

Studer dubbed his approach "hardwiring excellence," a metaphor fit for digital times and especially for Vanderbilt, which just then was also embarked on a parallel strategy to bring computer technology to bear on both research and patient care through informatics.[29] It also fit the style of Vanderbilt's management, who had already charted a business path for the institution little different from the best for-profit corporations, a path along which financial incentives drove behavior and results were measured endlessly and publicly.

The idea of a managerial scorecard was certainly not new with Studer, and the 2003 book, *Hardwiring Excellence*, added new categories and techniques. That was not the end of the process however. It began with the assumption that for people to deliver quality health care they must be highly self-motivated to do so, and they would be so only if their employer ministered to their most fundamental needs as workers.[30] Studer identified these needs as purpose, worthwhile work, and making a difference. Studer pictured his healthcare program as a "flywheel," to illustrate how an organization might accelerate change by turning the "passion" of employees (one arrow) into actions guided by key principles of service and operational excellence (the second arrow) that in turn achieved bottom line financial results (the third arrow). As it became clear how daily actions connected to core values at the hub of the flywheel (purpose, worthwhile work, making a difference, the needs behind self-motivation) and drove better performance, the wheel spun faster building momentum. Or as Studer put it, mixing his images, "success spirals upward."[31]

The flywheel figure was particularly fortuitous for Vanderbilt, where the medical center then had its own flywheel-like logo to distinguish it from the academic arm of the university.[32] Indeed, the two graphics were virtually identical but for the labeling. The translation of Studer's flywheel to Vanderbilt's was seamless and encouraged a sense that here was a believable approach to organizational change that was both bracing and affirmative. It was central to Studer's creed that most health care workers were idealists, but that bad systems blocked their way to high performance. Within any particular organization, certainly within Vanderbilt, it was equally important to be able to reinvigorate bedrock virtues with fresh resources of manifestation. Studer's highly instrumental "Pillars and Principles" approach provided it.

The "pillars," an idea that Studer had borrowed and adapted from Clay Sherman's 1993 book *Creating the New American Hospital: A Time for Greatness*, were meant to provide the categories for measurement against which all leaders would be evaluated and to help the organization balance short- and long-term goals. "Service," "Quality," "People," "Finance," and "Growth" were the headings that quickly rose to the top of Vanderbilt's corporate glossary. None was new. What *was* new was seeing them consciously expressed as both the foundational and aspirational heart of the Vanderbilt culture. In this case, "pillars," which both support and soar, were an apt image. Moreover, the pillars supported the structure together not separately, with improvement (or lack of it) under any one pillar sooner or later evident under all the others. Everything had a cause-and-effect relationship, and for better or worse everything showed in bottom line results.[33]

The "principles" simply provided the roadmap for reaching goals articulated under each of the pillars.[34] Studer likened the step-by-step process to a clinical pathway that moves toward a desired end, which although one of common sense, was, as he liked to add, "uncommonly practiced." "Committing to Excellence" meant setting goals or identifying desired results. "Measurement" was meant to align leadership and employee behavior. "Building a service culture" meant prescribing actions that would drive results and using "service teams" to connect values to actions. "Creating leaders" meant not only raising up leaders, but also developing them through distinct phases of organizational change. "Focusing on employee satisfaction" sought to liberate the idealism that moved people to enter the health care field and live it out on a daily basis. "Building accountability" meant to create a sense of "ownership" up and down the organization, demonstrating that the power of individual actions was visibly aligned with the actions of all individuals. "Owners," in Studer parlance, were accountable parties; "renters" were not.

Uniting behavior with goals meant developing measurable leadership evaluation tools—the all-important scorecard—and then holding leaders accountable for the results it revealed. "Communicating at all levels" meant constantly cascading information through the breadth and depth of the organization, on the assumption that no one individual alone could connect all the dots all the time. While hierarchy was inevitable, the organization had to be made to feel democratic lest it catch the "we/they" disease. Finally, "recognizing success" meant taking notice, calling attention, thanking people, and never growing complacent, in the belief that rewarded behavior replicates itself, multiplies, and creates more agreement and results, so accelerating the "flywheel."

The Studer approach went over well with the medical center's most distinguished scientists and clinicians as well as with its least skilled and educated employees. It suited an already numbers-driven management culture and supplied the tools to push that behavior downward through the organization to the point where it began to surge back up. And it addressed three critical institution-specific needs that the executive leadership believed were necessary to strengthen and sustain market leadership and business growth. It tackled, quantitatively, the question of what it meant to be a good employee, whether a dean, department head, or dishwasher. At its loftiest academic levels, Vanderbilt had long made great claims for its "collegiality." At humbler levels, among the mass of employees who worked for modest wages and the prospect of a pension, the need to belong and to know how to behave in order to belong was no less great. The pillars/principles/credo approach established a credible belief system accessible to all.

In time, a three-part institutional credo was elaborated with six enabling behaviors, all percolated through the Studer process: "I make those I serve my highest priority"; "I respect privacy and confidentiality"; "I communicate effectively"; " I conduct myself professionally"; "I have a sense of ownership"; "I am committed to my colleagues." To illustrate these behaviors, Vanderbilt devised a pillar on which these six statements were superimposed, the pillar's crown topped by the word *elevate*, by which word the ongoing program would become known. For the "V" in "elevate," designers cleverly situated the medical center's own circular three-arrow logo with the "V" at its center. (Or was that the Studer flywheel?)

Top to Bottom

"Transformation is not stamping out fires, solving problems, nor cosmetic improvements." That had been the judgment of W. Edwards Deming, the statistician and putative father of the modern quality movement, who in the 1950s first taught the idea of quality-as-system to managers and engineers in Japan. "Transformation," he asserted, "must be led by top management."[35]

Deming was equally adamant that best efforts and the hardest work never suffice, any more than would new machines or digital gadgets. He recounted how he once lay in a hospital bed, appalled at the evidence of inefficiencies all about him. He wondered why, on a Saturday, that he would not receive his prescribed medication until Monday, why a registered nurse who no doubt had other duties was making beds, and why the "theft-proof" coat hangers in the closet defied easy use. What, he wondered, was the moral of all this? What did it teach? One answer, verging on the glib, was that "the superintendent of the hospital needs to learn something about supervision," meaning learning something about making changes in procedure and taking responsibility for them. "Talks between physicians and nurses, even with the head nurse, accomplish nothing. A physician cannot change the system. A head nurse cannot change the system. Meanwhile who would know? To work harder will not solve the problem. The nurses *couldn't* work any harder."[36]

Deming died in 1993, when the principles of process improvement and their application to health care delivery were still in the courtship stage. Although it had matured, the relationship would not be permanent until those who advanced would have taught it and lived amid the medical education system. The consternation experienced by the Virginia Mason host when explaining waiting rooms to his Japanese visitor merely indicated the entrenched habits of American health care, behaviors practiced for so long as to become both unremarkable and unobjectionable. To continue the automotive metaphor, it is not unlike the acres of unsold cars at dealers across the US, vast inventory that is little more than capital sitting idle, expensive byproducts of a wasteful and inefficient system of manufacturing and selling.

Waste destroys value, and if no buyers come or if they go elsewhere, then value falls to nil. Practitioners of a certain age will remember an old line from the glory days of cost-plus medicine, before DRGs, managed care, HMOs, the Affordable Care Act and, yes, the whole tangle of teams, processes, and evidence bases. Their response to would-be reformers and cost-cutters then—" Hey, careful now: your waste is my profit!"—now tempts a knowing, retrospective sneer. But it went to the heart of the larger issue common to those times and our own: Who executes the best? Who reliably delivers the best value? Process improvement is a large part of the answer. "Who is paying" misses the point. It is notable that the largest growth market for the Studer Group is in Canada, where payer mix is irrelevant. But efficiency and organizational effectiveness remain imperative in Canada as they do everywhere.[37] No matter who pays, the commanding issue should be what are they buying? What they are buying in the future must be of greater value, greater quality, and safer and easier to obtain than it is today. Only endless process improvement can make good on that delivery.

Time was when nearly everyone knew the definition of GNP (gross national product) as the sum of goods and services produced in a country in a given year. Goods, obviously, were things that were made, whether by craft or mass or lean production. Services, it was assumed, came about differently. They were performed, as in "acted-out," and therefore something that seemed naturally, even excusably, variable and subjective, their value harder to pin down and measure. So what is good service? Well, you know it when you get it and you miss it when you don't. Health care may be thought of, first and last, as an altruistic service. To regard health care differently—as a good—is not to deny its service aspect but to enhance the level of service it can perform. In light of the demonstrated power of process improvement to raise value in health care, just as it did in automobile manufacturing, the "good" of health care fulfills both meanings of the word: as something concrete that is made, and as something that represents the creation of economic value. The meanings are linked.

In order to remain a good of the second sort, the good of the first sort must be made to an ever higher standard, something that can happen only through means more reliable than merely "being better" or "working harder." Just as happened at Virginia Mason with the introduction the Toyota Production System, many doctors today still object that medicine is too much an art to be amenable to such techniques. Medical practitioners may occasionally possess the singular touch of the artist, but that does not make medicine an art. Whereas every true work of art is singular and unique, the delivery of health care is very nearly its opposite, governed by system, routine, and repetition. Uniqueness marks the demand side, not the supply side. No two patients are exactly alike. But we have learned ways to make the care they buy into something uniform, safe, of high quality and lasting value.

SIX

1919: Getting It Done Now

So much noise accompanies today's health care debates that it is hard to hear anything at all intelligibly. On the one hand, it might be said that today's dire state of affairs—to which the system of service described in this book is a response—is unprecedented, even unique in history. But this only indicates a short memory.

We are also told that the solutions to our allegedly unprecedented problems lie right in our laps, and all that is lacking is "the will" to embrace change and shape the future to our enlightened design.[1] If this were so, then it would seem we ought to be doing better, given the number of best-intentioned people who know what needs to be done. Since neither of these scenarios is advancing progress, perhaps it's time to turn down the volume on debate and listen more carefully. A little history might be helpful, because history frees us from the tyranny of the present. We study it in order to understand what futures might be possible. Consider two events from one critical year in history: 1919.

The year 1919 is most famous, or infamous, for the Versailles peace conference and the treaty that officially wound-up the great blood-letting known to us as World War I, but known then as the "Great War." The Versailles treaty contained a war-guilt clause that blamed Germany for the war and imposed on it harsh reparations. In addition, the treaty established a "league of nations" invested with the duty to prevent any such cataclysm from ever happening again. The future that subsequent history disclosed was one of several possibilities only imperfectly foreshadowed in 1919. For example, had the United States joined the League; Hitler might not have come to power; Britain and France *might* have pushed Germany back in the Rhineland in 1936 without a fight, and so forth. Or alternatively, an embittered Germany *might* have rearmed and set out to avenge the humiliation of Versailles, while weak-willed democracies, desperate to keep peace at any price, appeased the dictators. Or, there might have been something in between. With hindsight, we can analyze all possible futures after 1919 and see that it was the least desirable one that came to pass.

More local but equally epochal in its own right, a second event from 1919 offered up its own possible futures. That September, John D. Rockefeller, Sr. signed over securities to the General Education Board, ultimately a total of $61 million, signaling the complete commitment of one of the world's great fortunes to the cause of re-making American medical education and with it American medicine. It was the largest single benefaction in the history of philanthropy and still, nine decades later, one of the largest ever. The Carnegie Corporation and others soon joined in, pushing totals over the next quarter-century into the hundreds of millions. For this, one man—Abraham Flexner—could claim to have been both catalyst and architect, and of the future that subsequently unfolded he would be the primary author. Or so at least we can judge today.

But remember the earnest peacemakers at Versailles, who failed to establish conditions favoring their most desired outcome, and who consequently fumbled the future. Nor, in the Flexner instance, was the most desired future the necessary one. It was possible (and in fact it actually happened) that the bad old medical order was more or less summarily dispatched, and a shiny new one institutionalized firmly in its place, with medical schools, and in time academic health centers filled with star physician-scientists. Or alternatively, the Flexner who had proven so brilliant a muckraker *might* have failed as Flexner the foundation-master and manager. He *might* have fumbled the execution of what he had so brilliantly keynoted back in 1910. He *might* have failed to find the right allies or enough of them. He *might* have fallen short of his patrons' high expectations and failed to sustain their commitment. Or alternatively yet, science itself *might* have faltered and failed to sustain its promise for medicine, one so evident to the men and women of Flexner's generation.

History should teach us at least this: an outcome that looks plausible, even inevitable, in retrospect is, after all, just one of numerous possibilities. "Reform" indeed seemed the obvious path to many of the most enlightened in medicine in 1919, but then so did peace seem the obvious path to the statesmen and diplomats at Versailles. And so we study the history for clues. We look back on certain events of 1919 and the future that followed, in order to learn of war and peace and of democracy's fragility and the dangers of appeasement—all matters still much with us today. We look back on other events of 1919 in order to learn how transformative change once came to medicine and under what conditions, and how it might do so again.

So we return to Abraham Flexner, the Louisville schoolmaster who a century ago burst on an antiquated and sclerotic medical scene, one beset by faulty incentives and pervasive inefficiencies—as it was then, so it is now. Flexner was no original thinker, but no one knew better how to implement other people's bright ideas and amplify their impact. Now as then, the right ideas clearly are available and all the stakeholders are eager to implement them. Yet nothing remotely comparable to Flexner's accomplishment—specifically, the comprehensive reform of American medical schools and medical care—is near at hand. The tools of course have changed. But the central problem that Flexner pressed so urgently to solve then—applying science to medicine in order to improve the standard of medical practice, and perhaps even to improve health—is still with us today.

Flexner would not have been able to do what he did without conviction in the belief that science in medicine was, at that moment, on the cusp of great things and that the age-old dream of medicine as a positive influence on human health could be realized. Although not a doctor, Flexner was on close terms with the greatest medical men of his age—Osler, Welch, Cushing, Robinson—and he yielded to no one in admiration for them. He saw the field of medical knowledge growing ineluctably and opening up, as he put it with typical economy in his famous report, "to quick, intelligent and effective action" as never before in its long, dreary history. "Provided, of course," he cautioned, "that the physician is himself competent to use the instrumentalities that have been developed! There is now the rub."

"Society reaps at this moment but a small fraction of the advantage which current knowledge has the power to confer," Flexner wrote prophetically. "That sick man is relatively rare for whom actually all is done that is at this day humanly feasible—as feasible in the small hamlet as in the large city, in the public hospital as in the private sanatorium."[2] That was in 1910, and it is still "the rub" in 2015.

For ideas to yield results, someone must be empowered to act. Ideas lying all about as they are today but applied piecemeal, waste their brilliance. Only if bundled up and made into the pillars of new institutions can they uphold a vision that will last through time. How Flexner bundled them then may help us to bundle them now.

Remembering What Flexner Did Then

Context is critical. By later measures, the load of cultural expectation on medicine in Flexner's lifetime was featherweight. The language then as yet contained no such concept as "health care" and certainly no notion of a positive "right" to it. There was little third-party insurance, private or public. There was little public support for research. But there was this: evidence enough that inductive science, applied to the study of human biology and the practice of medicine, promised (however faintly) to do things that medical men since antiquity had yearned to be able to do but had been powerless to achieve. The possibility beckoned of finally bringing down the curtain on the narrative of therapeutic desolation that was, relatively speaking, the story of medicine until that second half of the nineteenth century. It was hard to imagine a more virtuous, even thrilling prospect. Sinclair Lewis's *Arrowsmith* or A. J. Cronin's *The Citadel*, great medical novels from that era, capture the feeling. As possibility became probability, the medical profession was able to wrap itself in a mantle of authority and prestige unknown to it before. At long last, medicine worked, at least most of the time. And it worked because those who ruled its commanding heights and controlled its provision—MDs trained uniformly in curative medicine to Flexnerian standards—increasingly knew what they were doing and performed competently. Fewer doctors who were better doctors equaled better medicine.

In 1910, there were 150-plus medical schools in the United States, enrolling some 22,000 doctors-to-be, while the population of the country was 92 million.[3] Between what many of these institutions professed and the quality of the product they turned out lay a chasm at least as wide as today's disconnect between dollars spent on health care and actual health returned. It was that gap that Flexner's report documented and mercilessly excoriated. The report also found praiseworthy pockets of reform, such as Harvard, Michigan, Pennsylvania, and Hopkins where uncompromising high standards winnowed unfit institutions and established a new principle that quality not quantity of doctors was all that mattered. The standards become legend and iron-clad: two and preferably four years of college required for admission; a four-year course of study consisting of two years of pre-clinical basic science work followed by two years of clinical work; hospitals controlled by university administrations through full-time faculty, financing by endowment and expunging of any ves-

The Flexner Maps

ACTUAL DISTRIBUTION OF MEDICAL SCHOOLS

• Complete school   + Half-school
When two parts of a divided school are in close proximity
to each other, they are represented by one dot.

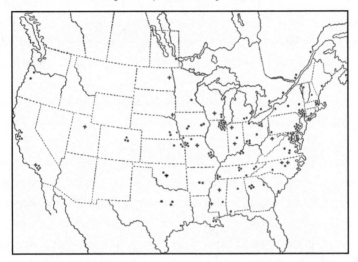

RECOMMENDED DISTRIBUTION OF MEDICAL SCHOOLS

• Complete school   + Half-school
When two parts of a divided school are in close proximity
to each other, they are represented by one dot.

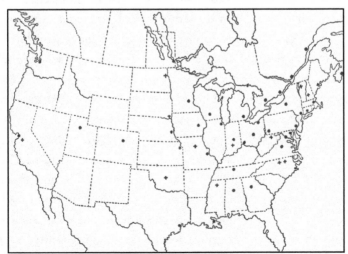

Source: Medical Education in the United States and Canada
(The Flexner Report), 1910.

tige of the profit motive. Flexner laid out a roadmap for reconstruction. The total number of medical schools shrank dramatically, with the surviving schools strategically distributed in large cities with a few in smaller towns, and graduating just half the doctors turned out in 1910. The sheer muckraking force of his report scared some proprietary schools into closing their doors overnight. Others would soon melt away.[4] "Factories for the Making of Ignorant Doctors" shouted headlines in the *New York Times* setting the general tone of high dudgeon at Flexner's exposé[5]—and setting the stage for more systematic change to come.

Remembering How Flexner Did It Then

Flexner drew attention not because of his originality—much of what he suggested was taken from current practices at Johns Hopkins and the German university system—but because of his ability to secure investment on a scale massive enough to be truly transformative and then to manage that investment in order to focus and condition its dispersal.

Critically, not every school needing help would get it. To attempt to assist all would have diluted investment so as to make it virtually useless. Rather, the new money would target a selection of frankly elite schools, in order to assure results so striking as to make them undisputed objects of emulation. Other schools, if they were in earnest about reform, would rise to the challenge of a transformed environment and find the resources to do the job on their own. Flexner had no doubt about this, even though it might take some time; America was even then a very rich country, and he knew the money was out there. Emulators in fact had no other viable choice. For years, weak, largely proprietary schools had been fading away unlamented, a warning of their fundamental insufficiency. Stronger ones, provided the right local leadership, could learn to survive and compete. And this was how it turned out to be.

The 1919 plan by which Flexner foresaw all this and thereby convinced potential investors bears some unpacking. He envisioned a core of high-quality, regionally organized medical institutions, and a second tier beneath them, which together would assure the country of the optimum supply of physician-scientists equipped both to serve the sick and to serve the cause of advancing medical understanding through science.

If ever proof were needed that large sums of money spent in service to the idea that progress meant strengthening the institutional structure of medical schools, then alignment of the Rockefeller philanthropies with medical education reform in the 1920s and 1930s provided it.[6] When in 1919, the Rockefellers committed to deep support of medical education, they were guided by Flexner's stipulation that careful selective subsidy would in the long run deliver greater impact than broader dispersal to many needy supplicants. Hammering away endlessly with signature phrases like "the modern ideal," "a modern basis of teaching," and "the highest-type medical school," Flexner sold his patrons on the need to build beacons, rather to aim for across-the-board standardization.

The Early Rockefeller Gifts[10]

DATE	INSTITUTION	TOTAL RAISED	ROCKEFELLER $	OTHER $
1913	Johns Hopkins	1,400,000	1,400,000	0
1914	Johns Hopkins	400,000	400,000	0
1919	Johns Hopkins	1,000,000	400,000	600,000
1914–19	Yale Univ	2,500,000	582,000	1,917,000
1914	Washington Univ	1,500,000	1,000,000	500,000
1919	Washington Univ	300,000	150,000	150,000
1916	Univ of Chicago	5,300,000	2,000,000	3,300,000

Source: "Medical Education in the United States: A Program,"
June 1919, Flexner Papers, Library of Congress.

Flexner laid out how it was to happen. In the nine years since 1910, the number of medical schools had fallen to ninety, and he predicted that more would soon disappear "through natural causes in the near future.[7] Eventually, he envisioned the Rockefeller money going to far fewer than that. Just thirty-one schools—from Baltimore, Philadelphia, New York, New Haven and Boston to Nashville and New Orleans, to Chicago, Iowa City, Cincinnati and St. Louis to Salt Lake City, San Francisco, and Seattle—would be enough, he said, to supply the country with an adequate stock of the "modern type" of doctor.[8]

A few of these institutions already possessed promising critical mass of talent to build upon, which made them appear obvious targets for investment. Indeed, the very top tier already had been. With the more modest funds available to the General Education Board before 1919, the largest share of support had gone to Hopkins, Washington University, Yale, and Chicago: about $8 million in all with much of it conditioned on local matching, largely aimed at replacing local practitioner-teachers with well-trained scientific faculty and (again, first and most famously at Hopkins) to establish clinical as well as basic science teaching on a "full-time university" basis.[9]

While there were controversies over the definition of "full-time university," Flexner maintained an unbending defense of its purity, even in the face of opposition from Sir William Osler, formerly of Hopkins and by then Regius Professor of Medicine at Oxford, Arthur Dean Bevan in Chicago, and Henry Christian and Harvey Cushing at Harvard. Flexner believed in an absolute separation of the new medical order, with its emphasis on scientific ideals, from the old one where practitioners too often seemed more obsessed with money-making. (At Columbia, Flexner made a particularly strong play, calling for the unification of the medical school and the Presbyterian hospital on a single site and for university control of hospital appointments and clinical "full-time." He sweetened the deal with $3 million from Rockefeller and Carnegie sources and ultimately succeeded over the opposition of Columbia president Nicholas Murray Butler.)

It was with the second tier of targets, however, that we see how reform played out across the continent and how, amid diverse local conditions, Flexner demonstrated a willingness to be flexible in order to get what he wanted. Flexner recognized that, as he wrote to John D. Rockefeller, Jr., the "proper educational procedure [must] be followed in the training of physicians who can apply such knowledge as has been won and who can utilize their current experience for the increase of knowledge and skill," but it did not follow that "uniform realization of an ideal type of medical school" was feasible quickly. Change was not possible at the same rate at every school, and new funds would most wisely be spent, Flexner argued, if employed "for the immediate *improvement* rather than the immediate *standardization* of medical education in the United States."[11]

He thought the Northeast likely to develop most quickly schools of the "highest type" and that "inasmuch as the Board cannot possibly cover the entire field," its benefaction there should go exclusively to those institutions that were the very best already, although with the understanding that there should be co-financing local resources). Institutions omitted from the benefaction would have to develop their own resources.

The South was a different matter, still, ninety years ago, very much the nation's domestic poor relation. The inputs, he judged, from the section's secondary schools and colleges could not yet reliably meet the requirements of modern medical schools. With the exception of his special project in Nashville at Vanderbilt, "which will be a constant source of inspiration and stimulus," he advised judicious help for existing schools with good potential in Virginia, Georgia, Texas, Louisiana, and elsewhere, which even though they fell short of the Nashville model were "susceptible of considerable improvement." The message was where the core was weak, then help those carefully at the margins, and be patient. The situation in the West raised an additional nuance of the probable need to help publicly-supported state universities, whereas the Board's experience thus far in medical education, in the East, had only been with private ones.

Flexner calculated methodically what it would all cost. For the first two (laboratory) years, he figured that an income of $100,000 would be sufficient to provide "modern teaching and research opportunities" for a student body of 250. Buildings and laboratories could be furnished with about $500,000. The clinical years were more difficult because of the need to build and maintain a hospital with a provision for teaching and research. Experience thus far had suggested that construction of a small, modern medical school with a hospital would run about $1 million and could be maintained with an endownment of an additional $1 million. A school of 250 students, then, needed an income of $200,000 for "current maintenance," of which fees would cover around $40,000. The balance would therefore require an endowment of $3 million, yielding income at 5 percent (aside from investment in physical plant and separate hospital endowment).[12]

The total cost of facilities and endowment per school Flexner put at a minimum of $6 to $7 million, with some schools needing much more if servicing large centers of population or prosecuting more elaborate forms of research. Thirty schools then meant $200 million total to do the job, and if half of those were to be more highly developed, as he believed they should be, then the sum would likely exceed $300 million.

The "Obtaining the Money" section of Flexner's June 1919 report, on behalf of the General Education Board to John D. Rockefeller, Sr., explained the disposition of these sums. Although the sums looked daunting, Flexner pointed out how the status of medical education had shifted from a "private business venture on the part of doctors" precluding philanthropic interest, to high-grade educational institutions under university auspices, a shift that changed the terms of engagement. Philanthropic benefaction, which had long been applied on behalf of college and university endowments now could be enlisted in the cause of medical institutions. The Rockefellers' first foray down this road had come with gifts of $1.8 million to the medical school and hospital of Johns Hopkins University in 1913 and 1914. But it was in the power of such singular benefaction to attract yet other resources that Flexner saw as the key to meeting the challenge. "Medical schools of university grade are more and more acquiring the status of colleges and universities," Flexner noted, "so that large sums may be raised through the leverage of [Rockefeller] gifts representing an important, though in many cases not the preponderating, share in the undertaking." Doubtless, the terms on which progress could be made would become more favorable, he added, "as the movement gained in momentum and public recognition."[13] He was certainly right about that. From 1914 to 1919, Hopkins, Yale, Washington University, and the University of Chicago raised, in aggregate, $10.6 million for medical education reform, of which $3.7 million came from Rockefeller sources, with the balance from outside. (See chart above.)

Flexner compared the requirements of the medical challenge with previous contributions to general university endowment ($15 million since 1906) and emphasized that the Rockefellers, if they were in earnest about championing this cause, would need to raise considerably more than that. But if they did, he argued, then the proven power of leverage (except perhaps in the relatively poor South where local resources would likely be slim for some time come) was sure to take hold. He was not shy, and in general he was correct: "If a fund of say $30 million [and the Rockefellers alone ultimately came in for more than $60 million] were available, principal and interest to be distributed within a period varying from twenty-five to fifty years, it seems by no means improbable that, partly through its leverage and partly through the momentum thus communicated to medical education, a total sum of two hundred millions could be added to the resources of the thirty-one schools required to satisfy the country's needs." Flexner's persuasion worked, and the Rockefeller philanthropies stepped up. By the end of the 1920s, out of sixty-four medical schools still in operation in the United States, forty percent, or twenty-five, received Rockefeller support.[14] The result was dramatic beyond even the numbers. What had occurred was the replacement of the pre-1910 jumble of weak institutions varying in quality with a loosely coordinated but functionally uniform system of schools and associated hospitals.[15] Their impact was to make clinical medicine into a scientific discipline and to instill a standard of excellence that would govern the ethos of the medical profession, as well as academic medicine, for a century and counting.

The reformed "system" came about, then, by a process of judicious selection and categorical support that Flexner controlled almost singlehandedly. In essence, he went into partnership with those he deemed the most promising entrepreneurial deans and university presidents, who were also exceptional fundraisers. Together, they worked out the details of bringing the new order of medical education to their select institutions. He was pushy, demanding, uncompromising, and almost always got his way. Most often, this meant improving already-exemplary institutions and leveraging the power of their example to schools beyond the scope of Rockefeller largesse in order to inculcate in them the drive to "take care of themselves."[16]

Two examples stand out of a different model where Flexner advised something more radical. Subsequent history confirmed that it was possible—in the right conditions, perhaps even preferable—to begin again virtually from scratch. Vanderbilt University, in the early twentieth century a small, provincial school in Nashville, received $13 million from the Rockefellers' General Education Board (with an additional grant from Carnegie) on the condition that it *start all over again* with its medical school. Its old school had strong but thin local medical leadership, and practically no modern facilities. But it was at Vanderbilt that Flexner found in James H. Kirkland one of his greatest-ever academic allies, and the sort of leader with whom he could conspired to conjure something from almost nothing. Together, they imported the very best new talent, starting at the top with G. Canby Robinson, student of Osler and resident physician at Simon Flexner's research institute in New York City, a young man who was even pushier (if that was possible) than Abraham Flexner. Robinson came to Vanderbilt from the deanship at Washington University in St. Louis, which had been one of the targets of the first round of Rockefeller grants. The Vanderbilt grant, as Flexner vividly put it, "acted like a depth bomb" across the region, demonstrating clearly how other schools would have to exert themselves in order to survive.[17]

In upstate New York meanwhile, the University of Rochester had had no medical school at all, a deficit on which Flexner capitalized with vigor. With Columbia and Cornell in New York City moving slower than he wished toward full-time clinical teaching, Flexner saw in the then relatively remote school in western New York the rare chance to create a "medical school of the modern type" truly *de novo*. Not only did the University of Rochester possess a president of outstanding leadership, Rush Rhees, the region was also home to local Kodak magnate and philanthropist George Eastman. Eastman put in $5 million of the $10 million total, an increase inveigled at length by the inexhaustible Flexner, whom Eastman referred to as "the worst highwayman that ever flitted into and out of Rochester. He put up a job on me and cleaned me out of a thundering lot of my hard-earned savings."[18]

The result, both at Rochester and Vanderbilt, were new, purpose-built, functionally-coordinated physical plants integrating hospitals, laboratories, and teaching spaces, all populated with fresh intellectual capital that made those institutions true models for their times. Moreover, the philanthropy that enabled their creation was as heavily conditioned as it was bounteous. It was not offered and was not allowed to be spent piecemeal—no "cracked ice" as the Rockefeller Foundation's Alan Gregg famously described the low impact of small grants. The aim was not just "reform" but creation of powerful new institutions, which both Vanderbilt and Rochester literally were. Nothing less than transformative investment could have raised them up from near nothing. Nothing less would do.

Partial Resurrection

A century later, the Carnegie Foundation for the Advancement of Teaching produced a sequel to the Flexner Report. Commissioned in 2004 and published in 2010, *Educating Physicians: A Call for Reform of Medical School and Residency* was a team effort, rather than a solo act as had been Flexner's original. The 2010 report belonged to a larger Carnegie-sponsored project to evaluate the state of professional education in several fields including lawyers, engineers, clergy, and nurses.[19] Its authors admitted that their report stood proudly on Flexner's model, in particular, his key technique of *ambulando discimus*, "learning by walking around" (with which every medical student and resident physician remains familiar to this day). Flexner personally had "walked around" all of the then-155 medical schools in the United States and Canada, a feat that the modern team did not attempt to replicate. Their brief was different: not exposing the bad but gathering up examples of the most innovative and, on that basis, distilling recommendations for the future. They visited only fourteen institutions, chosen because of their "interesting educational innovations" and representing a variety of institutional types and different geographical regions.[20]

Educating Physicians made four broad recommendations for the future of medical education. To educate doctors in ways that comprehend contemporary changes in medical practice, in therapeutic intervention and the technologies available to medicine, and in the competencies and processes required to master them will require, it declared: 1) standardizing of learning outcomes while individualizing learning processes; 2) integrating formal knowledge with clinical experience; 3) instilling habits of inquiry and continuous improvement that will make the doctor's education a lifelong one; and 4) instilling a profound professional identity.[21] Much as Flexner had steeped himself in fresh ideas about progressive education and the ideas of John Dewey, the new report's conclusions drew on the latest educational research in the learning sciences and (inevitably) reflected the cultural and economic anxieties of its times.

In any case, the primary issue is no longer, as it was for Flexner and his generation, the reform of medical education from which would then flow naturally, it was thought in those simpler times, better medicine. The central issue now is bridging the gap between discovery and health by innovating in service delivery—the great black hole into which so much of today's best-intentioned "reforms" ingloriously tumble. Bridging the gap and that alone will bring to reality the system of service whose components we have described in the preceding chapters of this book (and of which medical education reform, as advocated in *Educating Physicians* and elsewhere, is understood to be a part). Finding and applying means to do this is the unique challenge of our moment in history, yet it is analogous to the problem Flexner faced.

For the difference between then and now we can only blame success. Our challenge is bigger and more complex because medicine now is so much better than it was then. By "better" we mean "more expensive." It is because, in between the sick and their healers, between patients and their physicians, has grown up a jungle of contentious third parties. It is because medicine, once understood as a professional sometimes charitable service, has morphed into health care delivered as a consumable commodity and claimed as a positive right—a shift in behavior and expectation that drives demand beyond any conceivable capacity to satisfy it.[22]

"Revolutionary ideas" (or the even more overused "new paradigms") are rare, the result of changes long building under the right catalysts. Flexner caught a wave of evolutionary change in medicine that had been gathering force in North America and Europe for at least half a century. Evolution became revolution, however, for just one reason: Flexner's command of immense external resources. He sold—and "sold" is precisely the right verb—the leadership of great philanthropies on the worth and urgency of his cause and persuaded them that history would vindicate their support. Today, we stand where Flexner stood in 1910: the moment when all the ideas were on the table but before the resources were committed. Today, we need to reach our own "1919 moment." Where the resources can come from now, and how they can be deployed so to be catalysts for the revolution that will close the gap between discovery and health is suggested below.

To all those who will seek to apply this template, history holds three points: 1) the necessity of focusing on a singular driving idea; 2) the necessity of concentrating effort and not spreading resources too thin; 3) the necessity of applying resources that are large enough to be transformative and then letting emulation do its work elsewhere. There is a fourth point—the necessity to measure outcomes—on which the history here is silent. While Flexner's generation lacked the tools to measure outcomes, the greater problem was that it simply did not occur to them that measurement might be necessary. To Flexner's contemporaries, better medical education made for better medical doctors which made for better medicine, and, it was assumed, better health. Somewhere between then and now, history interrupted that happy progress and pointed to more troubled times, which is where we live today. Measuring outcomes is the new necessity, and the tools are at hand.

The Additional Problem

It cannot be repeated too often—the degree to which Flexner's doings transformed medical education and institutionalized the union of science and medicine—because if we forget the history, we forfeit the power of analogy to teach. Thus, the challenge today: What are the decisive steps that we can take to transform our dismayingly dysfunctional health care delivery system and to institutionalize the translation of biomedical science into clinical practice, thus closing the gap between what we know and what we do? The chapters above describe the system of service that it must be our goal to meet. To bring this about, however, and to move from advocacy to action, requires lifting some operational pages from Flexner's book and applying them to the remaining obstacle blocking our path: a health-care service industry that is resistant to innovation.

"Give us the tools," Winston Churchill famously put it to the American president and people in February 1941 when Britain was still fighting alone, "and we will finish the job!" Science is providing us with the tools to win more and larger victories over sickness and suffering, and in all likelihood it will continue to do so at an ever-increasing pace—drugs vetted through well-designed clinical trials, all manner of diagnostic devices, molecular and genetic insights, an ever-more authoritative evidence base. But before we can finish the job, the health care service industry must be supplied with its own new tools if it is to take responsibility for delivering the right care to the right patient at the right time in the right setting. This means applying science to clinical practice with far greater efficiency then we do now. To maintain and restore health at an affordable cost (that is, to achieve better outcomes faster and cheaper) is to create social, scientific, and, not least, economic value. For this to happen, serious reform and innovation in service delivery is imperative. This will seem no less daunting than the reforms Flexner contemplated in his day, and now as then, it will require singular vision and serious investment. But if it is pursued with determination, and if in the end it is successful, the return on the investment will be huge.

As we have pointed out before, most efforts to influence the relentlessly rising cost of health care have focused on changing how we pay for it, who pays for it, and how much. This has proven a dead end. Fiddling with payment methodology and jiggering reimbursement rates have not slowed the growth of per capita spending on health care in the US, nor have they produced a safer delivery system with measurably superior outcomes. The focus of reform must shift from how we pay for health care to what it is we are buying.

Health care, it is endlessly said, is impossibly complex. But it need not be a complete mystery. Everything that we are buying can be better understood and more clearly grappled with when organized into a short series of related but functionally distinct tasks.[23] To each, we can assign a numerical grade for how well the U.S. health care system performs. We acknowledge that there are isolated pockets of superior performance across all these tasks, but the grades we have assigned are meant to reflect overall performance. It is not a happy picture.

The nine tasks include screening; prevention; education and behavior modification; provision of routine care (largely an outpatient activity); delivery of serious acute care (largely an inpatient service necessitated by such clinical conditions as serious trauma, acute heart attack or stroke, organ transplantation, etc.); management of chronic illness (the 20 percent of the population that account for 80 percent of our health care expenditures); rehabilitation (restoring individuals to maximum functionality whether they have had a joint replacement, a heart attack or stroke, an exacerbation of chronic obstructive pulmonary disease, or a serious bout of depression); elder care (selected as a separate task because of the aging demographic of the US population and because of the high disease burden of this population); and, finally, end of life care (up to 25 percent of our health care resources are expended on individuals in their last year of life). If a grade of five or at least four is the target, then we are woefully underperforming in seven of these nine essential jobs.

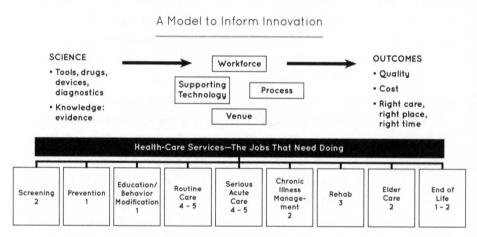

A Model to Inform Innovation

Performance: 5 = Outstanding; 1 = Poor

It is not hard to select any clinical problem or public health issue or disease category and inquire what tools science has provided to address them and what the evidence base has provided as a guideline for the application of these tools. The answers to these two questions (which is "quite a lot" in both cases) then however call for execution, which historically we do not do well. Execution means the optimal integration of four ingredients: 1) the appropriate workforce (physicians, nurses, pharmacists, social workers, dieticians, technicians, family members, case managers); 2) the processes employed by this workforce; 3) the appropriate venues where the work is to be performed (hospital, clinic, rehabilitation center, home, nursing home, workplace, pharmacy, storefront clinics); and 4) the supporting technology (information technology, remote sensing, telemedicine).

People, Process, Venue, Technology

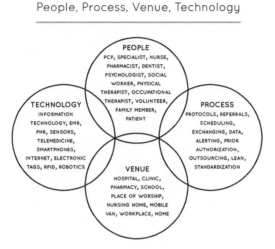

Consider the example of breast cancer to see the promise and the broad applicability as well as the pervasive gaps in how we now go about delivery of care. Has science and the evidence base provided us tools and direction in how to screen for breast cancer? Yes. What about prevention and patient education? Again, yes. Routine care, yes. There are good guidelines for follow-up of an abnormal screening mammogram. For serious acute care? Effective radical mastectomy. For chronic illness management? Yes, there are good protocols for recurrent conditions and for rehabilitation after mastectomy or reconstructive surgery. For end of life? Here, the answer is another question: should this disease all too often still be fatal? Let us check how our current system performs on the key job of screening in breast cancer. As documented by Jack Wennberg and his group in the Dartmouth Atlas, screening for breast cancer is highly variable across the country. Wennberg was able to determine using Medicare data what percent of women received adequate breast cancer screening. Dividing the country into more than 300 Medicare markets, Wennberg found that women in Traverse City, Michigan, were screened at about half the rate they should have been, whereas women in Columbia, South Carolina, were screened at only a 19 percent rate. It is a tragic commentary on how we fail to execute on the evidence base. At best, in breast cancer screening, we are doing the right thing half the time. We have the tools. We know what we should do. Yet, we do not get it right. This 50 percent performance metric (in layman's terms, we might just as well call it the failure rate) is hardly limited to breast cancer screening. In a study by the Rand Corporation, researchers evaluated whether patients who lived in twelve northeastern cities received evidence-based care for a range of both acute health issues and for chronic conditions. In both cases, the right care was provided a bit more than half the time.[24]

The Gap Between What We Know and What We Do

6,712 individuals in 12 cities
    Only 54.9 percent received recommended care
    Only 54.9 percent received recommended preventive care
    Only 53.5 percent received recommended acute care
    Only 56.1 percent received recommended chronic care

Examples:	Hip fracture	22.8 percent
		(range 6.2–39.5 percent)
	Atrial fibrillation	24.7 percent
	Depression	57.2 percent
	Senile cataract	78.7 percent (best performance)

Source: E. A. Glynn, et al., *New England Journal of Medicine*, June 26, 2003.

It is clear that our system of care has a serious execution problem and that attempts to influence its performance by modifying the approach to payment have not delivered meaningful results. In another Rand study of approaches to value-based purchasing, precious little evidence for scalable transformation of care delivery could be identified. Commissioned by the Office of the Assistant Secretary for Planning and Evaluation in Health and Human Services, the study evaluated 129 value based purchasing (VBP) programs. Ninety-one were pay for performance (P4P) program, 27 were Accountable Care Organizations (ACOs), and 11 were Bundled Payment (BP) programs. Also, Rand evaluated the peer-reviewed published literature and convened a Technical Expert Panel (TEP) of payors, providers, sponsors of VBP programs, and health service researchers to which Rand provided the summary of the environmental survey and the literature review. This study, along with its companion report, "Measuring Success in Health Care Value—Based Purchasing Programs— Summary and Recommendations" are important, and depressing, reading.[25]

While the Rand study was thorough and comprehensive and identified both positive trends and shortcomings, still, over almost fourteen years of value-based purchasing experiments, it could not identify a significant impact of such programs on the quality or the cost of health care. The study concluded lamely: "There have been mixed feelings on the effectiveness of VBP programs to meet its intended goals to improve quality and control costs.... When we queried the Technical Expert Panel about the features of successful VBP programs based on their knowledge from having designed and operated these programs, most panelists agreed that the evidence is thin regarding successful programs and what features characterize these programs."

As is typical with so many such "silver bullets," there appears to be at least surface logic supporting value-based purchasing (along with bundled payments, another initiative being tested). Unfortunately, the vast majority of the provider community is simply not prepared, either structurally or operationally, to innovate practically on the basis of this kind of experiment. In the value-based purchasing strategy and related initiative, there is a fatal flaw, namely, the mistaken assumption that real innovation in service delivery can take place in an environment where the innovators are at financial risk, and do not have the resources, either human or financial, truly to innovate in care delivery. Program sponsors and supporters of such approaches are mistaken to think that an experiment in the context of a competitive market, involving providers who lack appropriate infrastructure and who struggle with thin financial margins, can possibly yield real innovation in care-execution. How could it be otherwise? On the contrary, the innovation required truly to reduce the gap between what we know and how we perform demands (in addition to a well-designed research protocol, broader performance targets and a goal of wholesale performance improvement) up-front investment. Chasing a financial reward for some limited set of improved outcomes is like "teaching to the test." This approach cannot hard-wire the kind of innovative change that comprehensively and consistently translates science into clinical practice.

So, do we continue to tinker with how we pay for health care, in hope that the delivery system will somehow re-invent itself? Or do we make a deliberate attempt at transforming the delivery of care through research-driven innovation in service-delivery, thereby shifting the focus onto what we it is we are buying?

We believe that our model of health care delivery that divides the necessary work into discrete modules can be used to design innovative solutions for much of what we currently do not do well. Using our model we can, as we demonstrate earlier, take a significant unmet need and ask what work in which models needs to be redesigned with a truly innovative approach. We are not talking just about creativity. Innovation requires creativity and execution.

We have spent enough time coming up with ideas that do not work, can not work, or are not executed. Innovation in service delivery requires first, identification of the customer (this is almost always a group of individuals with a given clinical condition). The innovation process then identifies the needs of the customer with special emphasis on the significant unmet needs (for example, Hemoglobin Alc normalization in Type II diabetics). Then, we turn to the model and created the solution by designing the best mix of people (the workforce), process, technology, and venue. In the example of Hgb Alc, we are working in the management of chronic disease module. Besides the physician, who in this clinical example should share accountability for achieving the goal, it is clear that nurse educations, dietitians, pharmacists, and the patient's family support must all play key roles. An electronic medical record with decision support, dashboards, and alerting capabilities is another must. Integration of mobile devices for communication (especially for texting), data transfer, coaching (diet, physical activity) and creation of patient communities are examples of necessary supporting technology. Management of such patients should require very few in person visits to a physician office or clinic. Using mobile technology as well as telemedicine should allow for management to be in any venue and to be both synchnous and asynchronous.

Today, almost 45 percent of diabetics have Hemoglobin Alc greater than 7 percent and 20 percent have Hemoglobin Alc of greater than 90 percent! Clearly the way we deliver care for this population is not coming close to desired outcomes. The cost in morbidity and mortality is enormous.

Flexner for Today

It is past time to begin again now, with the solution that fits this problem. History instructs us to embrace a program no less transformative than Flexner's, which succeeded not just because of its own internal brilliance but also because of its author's ability to convince the great philanthropists of that era to finance it. What would this program look like today and what could it accomplish?

Just as Flexner proposed an experiment with relatively few medical schools and a strategy that, if successful, would cause other schools to follow suit or fall away, we too propose an experiment with a select group of health care provider-institutions, no more than a dozen, both academic and community-based. Each will receive major multi-year research funding for the sole purpose of innovating in service delivery around the nine demand modules described earlier. The charge to these recipients will be to integrate people, process, technology and venue in order to improve the cost and quality of care for the entire population of patients they serve. Through their research efforts, these institutions must achieve a wholesale change in performance, not just a limited set of outcome measures or compliance with a list of processes. They must measurably improve population health, reduce morbidity and mortality even as they reduce per capita health-care spending.

None of this is remotely possible, of course, if we continue on our current path of touting innovation while failing to invest in it. No less than the process of discovery in basic science, real innovation in service delivery requires real research, and research takes real money. What then might such a transformative experiment and associated investment look like? How would the participating entities be selected? How much funding would be necessary and where would it come from? What kind of oversight and evaluation would be necessary and by whom?

Recall that Flexner's revolution surged forward on the strength of one initial, large investment: John D. Rockefeller's 1919 commitment of $61 million to support the transformation of medical education.[26] In today's dollars (factored as a percent of US GDP), this single commitment equals $13.6 billion. As large as it is, this sum simply would not get the job done today. Granting the need for further definition of the scope and duration of these research projects, it is our conviction that meaningful outcomes that could be scaled-up via the mechanism of emulation will take five to seven years of work by about a dozen entities sharing a total budget of $30 billion.

A large sum certainly, but insignificant when compared to the total dollars we will spend in this country on health care over a five to seven year period. (At $2.8 trillion per year, that would come to $14 to $20 trillion, of which $30 billion comes to less than one quarter of one percent.) Moreover, it is also trivial as a research and development budget, when we remember that pharmaceutical, biotechnology, and medical device companies routinely spend 10 to 15 percent of their revenue on product innovation, or research and development. Such comparison goes to the very heart of the challenge before us—and underscores the magnitude of our neglect in this key, indeed *the* key, health care sector, up to now. Health care service enterprises, whether academic medical centers, proprietary hospital chains, not-for-profit health systems, community hospitals or physician groups, have essentially nothing—yes, *nothing*—in their budgets dedicated to research in service delivery. Yet, this is the business they are in. By analogy, without public and private-sector R&D funding, sustained now over many decades, we would not have the biomedical science that today begs for better delivery. In order to translate this ever-increasing body of knowledge into clinical practice effectively and efficiently, comparable investment in service delivery innovation can be delayed no longer. The research that is necessary to drive this innovation will not just come about of its own accord. Rather, it must be intentionally designed, well-executed, and objectively-evaluated, and when valuable discoveries in service delivery result, they must be disseminated quickly and incorporated into practice by the broader health care service community.

Where then can a $30 billion, five-to-seven-year research budget come from? The United States is unique among other countries in the regulation, financing, and service-delivery domains of its health care system. We are very much a private/public blend, with service provision largely private and financing majority private but with a large and growing public (government) component. This pluralist heritage can be an advantage. It multiplies the responsible stakeholders who can plausibly be called upon to participate in financing service-delivery research and ultimately in reaping its rewards. We propose therefore that the Department of Health and Human Services (representing Centers for Medicare and Medicaid Services [CMS], NIH, and the FDA), the private health insurance industry, the pharmaceutical, biotechnology, medical device and diagnostics sectors, and the service-provider community shoulder responsibility and participate equally in funding this initiative. We do not believe $30 billion when spread over a minimum of five years among this number of stake-holders would be burdensome. Additionally, the return on investment (which is probably less risky than much basic science research has been in the past and still is) promises not to be trivial. For CMS and the private insurance industry, the return is obvious. Any successful research initiative in service-delivery inno-vation that can be scaled-up across the country would necessarily right-size and control the rate of growth of health-care spending—that holy grail of health-care policymakers that has forever been out of reach. As for the NIH and FDA, with their legacy interest in seeing science and the tools to which science has given birth translated into effective and safe clinical care, they could hardly be better served than by commensurate innovation (read "discovery") in service-delivery. Nothing could better amplify their mission to promote evidence-based applica-tion of scientific and clinical research and the products generated from it than to direct it to the daily benefit of patients. The health-care service industry itself stands to improve its performance, and possibly its financial viability and sus-tainability, through market adoption of innovative approaches to care delivery. Finally, and most importantly, by thus narrowing the gap between what we know and the tools we have and how we leverage them to maintain and restore health, we can bring immense and measurable benefit to the people we serve.

How would we organize, administer, and monitor such a bold initiative in health-care service research? Certainly not as Flexner did a century ago, or-ganizing his revolution in collboration with a few like-minded (some would say toadying) foundation heads, medical deans and university presidents. Such a unitary, command-and-control approach is no longer possible or desirable in this age of transparency and accountability. We recommend, rather, the cre-ation of a multi-discipline project-management group composed of appropriate individuals from those key organizations and entities with a commitment to improving the health of our population. These organizations would include The Centers for Medicare and Medicaid Services (CMS), The Agency for Health-care Research and Quality (AHRQ), The Institute of Medicine (IOM), The National Institutes of Health (NIH), and The Healthcare Leadership Council (HLC). Representatives from these organizations should create a working group to define all the major components of the research initiative we have sketched in this proposal: 1) defining the goals of the research, including a detailed set of outcome measures that will confirm whether or not resulting innovations can indeed significantly improve on population health and cost, as well as the ability of any particular service-delivery innovation to scale across the broad health-care service community; 2) creating a selection committee to establish the criteria for selecting the research sites; 3) defining precise mechanisms for funding the project, including the appropriate distribution of funding responsibility among the public and private sources identified above; and finally 4) defining the how and the whom of monitoring and evaluating research progress.

1919 Moment

To "begin again now," and in this way, is radical but also doable. Its analogue has happened before under different but no less challenging circumstances, and the record is there for our instruction. From our proposal—calling for nothing less than transformative-scale investment in leadership-worthy institutions the power of whose example can move the vast system—you may infer our judgment on the ceaseless noise of health-care reform referenced at the beginning of this chapter and this book. Reform up to and including the Affordable Care Act in all its iterations has failed, and will continue to fail, to deliver on the full promise that science in medicine still makes to mankind. As long as demand for the goods of medicine and health remain limitless, reform will perforce continue—and it will continue to fall short of the outcomes we desire even as it bankrupts the nation. We are not, to use the fashionable term, on a sustainable path.

We live in a world far from that of Flexner. Yet, even factoring out all the now-offensive differences from those bad old, elitist times, there remains something irreducible about that long-ago episode that needs no translation or qualification. Yesterday's "reformed system" came about only by a process of unapologetic selection and categorical support that Flexner controlled, if not quite singlehandedly then in closest partnership with those he deemed the most promising entrepreneurial deans and university presidents (and whose equivalents across a broader institutional spectrum await their call today).[27] Together, they then worked out the details of bringing the new order of medical education to their select institutions. Flexner was pushy, demanding, uncompromising, yes arrogant, and he almost always got his way. Most often, this meant improving the best existing institutions and leveraging the power of their example to those other schools beyond the scope of Rockefeller largesse but which nonetheless grasped the mandate and had the drive, in Flexner's phrase, to "take care of themselves."[28]

Just as those leaders did then, here is our chance to begin again—*now*. We invite all comers to join the process and fix with us upon this highest-value, yet wholly attainable goal. If the next Flexner steps forward from among you who are reading this, who can accomplish even half of what the original did, then our book will have served its purpose, and historians and policymakers a century hence may look back to this latter-day "1919 moment" for clues to how our generation got it done and began again—now.

NOTES

Preface: Where We Are and Why It Matters

1 See Charles Rosenberg, *Our Present Complaint: American Medicine Then and Now* (Baltimore, MD: Johns Hopkins University Press, 2007), 4–5.

History: Abraham Flexner's Dangerous Big Idea

1 Following, Proceedings of Abraham Flexner, a Tribute, National Fund for Medical Education, 1956, Vanderbilt University Medical Library.

2 Thomas Bonner, *Iconoclast: Abraham Flexner and a Life in Learning* (Baltimore, MD: Johns Hopkins University Press, 2002); Abraham Flexner, *I Remember* (New York, NY: Simon & Schuster, 1940), revised edition published in 1960 as *Abraham Flexner: An Autobiography*; Timothy C. Jacobson, *Making Medical Doctors: Science and Medicine at Vanderbilt Since Flexner* (Tuscaloosa, AL, and London, England: University of Alabama Press, 1987).

3 On the reform movement in medical education at the turn of the century, H. D. Banta, "Abraham Flexner—A Reappraisal," *Social Science Medicine* 5 (1971), 655–61; Howard S. Berliner, "A Larger Perspective on the Flexner Report," *International Journal of Health Sciences* 5 (1975), 573–92 and "New Light on the Flexner Report: Notes on the AMA-Carnegie Foundation Background," *Bulletin of the History of Medicine* 51 (1977), 603–09; Daniel M. Fox, "Abraham Flexner's Unpublished Report: Foundations and Medical Education, 1909–1928, *Bulletin of the History of Medicine* 54 (1980), 475–96; Robert P. Hudson, "Abraham Flexner in Perspective: American Medical Education, 1865-1910," *Bulletin of the History of Medicine* 46 (1972), 545–61; Henry Miller, "Fifty Years After Flexner," *Lancet* 2 (1966) 647–54; Saul Jarcho, "Medical Education in the United States, 1910–1956," *Journal of the Mt. Sinai Hospital* 8 (1959), 339–85.

4 Following, Jacobson, *Making Medical Doctors*, 31–52.

5 *The Flexner Report, Medical Education in the United States and Canada*, Bulletin Number 4, Carnegie Foundation for the Advancement of Teaching (1910), x.

6 *Ibid.*, 156.

7 One doctor for every 1,000 people in the cities, one for every 2,000 in rural areas, for an average ratio nationwide of 1:1,500. In America, the oversupply of poorly

trained doctors already in practice would diminish by attrition. By limiting production to one new doctor for every increase of 1,500 in the general population, he
believed that over the next generation the proper ratio could be established without
causing a shortage.

8 *The Flexner Report*, 48.

9 A sampling: *Medical Education: Final Report on the Commission on Medical Education* (AAMC, 1932); *Medical Education in the United States* (AMA, 1940); *Trends in
Medical Education* (The Commonwealth Fund, 1949); *Medical School in the United
States at Mid-Century* (AMA/AAMC, 1953); *Physicians for a Growing America* (United States Public Health Service, 1959); *Planning for Medical Progress through Education* (AAMC, 1965); *Medical Education Reconsidered* (American Surgical Association,
1966); *The Graduate Education of Physicians* (AMA, 1966); *Higher Education and the
Nation's Health: Policies for Medical and Dental Education* (Carnegie Commission on
Higher Education, 1970); *A Handbook for Change* (Student American Medical Association, 1972); *Future Directions for Medical Education* (AMA, 1982); *The New Biology and Medical Education: Merging the Biological, Information and Cognitive Sciences*
(Josiah Macy Foundation, 1983); *Physicians for the Twenty-first Century* (AAMC,
1984); *Healthy America: Practitioners for 2005* (Pew Health Professions Commission,
1991); *Improving Access to Health Care through Physician Workforce Reform* (United
States Public Health Service, 1992); *Medical Education in Transition* (Robert Wood
Johnson Foundation, 1992); *Education Medical Students: Assessing Change in Medical
Education, the Road to Implementation* (AAMC, 1992); *Health Professions Education
for the Future: Schools in Service to the Nation* (Pew Health Professions Commission,
1993).

10 Following, see Nicholas A. Christakis, "The Similarity and Frequency of Proposals
to Reform US Medical Education," *Journal of the American Medical Association
(JAMA)*, 274: 706–11, September 6, 1995.

11 *The Flexner Report*, 42.

12 The latest, also Carnegie-sponsored, fittingly appeared in the centennial year, 2010:
Molly Cooke et al, *Educating Physicians: A Call for Reform of Medical School and
Residency* (Stanford, CA: Carnegie Foundation for the Advancement of Teaching/
Jossey-Bass, 2010). See discussion, Chapter Six, below.

13 Christakis, 706, 711.

14 Samuel Bloom, "Structure and Ideology in Medical Education: An Analysis of Resistance to Change," *Journal of Health and Social Behavior* 29:294–306 (1988); also see

Renee C. Fox, "Time to Heal Medical Education," *Academic Medicine*, 74: 1072–75, October 1999.

15 For a spirited discussion of this past, see Ezekiel J. Emanuel, *Healthcare, Guaranteed: A Simple, Secure Solution for America* (New York, NY: Public Affairs, 2008), 41–80.

16 On this vexed question see for opposing arguments: Richard A. Epstein, *Mortal Peril: Our Inalienable Right to Health Care?* (Cambridge, MA: Perseus Books, 1999) and Jonathan Wolff, *The Human Right to Health* (New York, NY: W. W. Norton and Company, Inc., 2012).

17 Down in the trenches of daily practice, where patients matter more than politics, the ACA looked to many harried physicians and surgeons like little more than managed care on steroids.

One: Translating Discovery

1 Although they are not systematically incorporated into measures of national income. See William D. Norhaus, "The Health of Nations: The Contribution of Improved Health to Living Standards," Kevin D. Murphy and Robert H. Topel, eds., *Measuring the Gains from Medical Research: An Economic Approach* (Chicago, IL: University of Chicago Press, 2003), 9–40.

2 See Robert Fogel, "Economic Growth, Population Theory , and Physiology: The Bearing of Long-term Processes on the Making of Economic Policy," *American Economic Review* (June 1994).

3 *Ibid.*

4 Murphy and Topel, "The Economic Value of Medical Research," 41–73.

5 Frank R. Lichtenberg, "Pharmaceutical Innovation, Mortality Reduction and Economic Growth," 74–109.

6 In 2000, the US government-funded $18.4 billion for medical research, European Union $3.7 billion.

7 Although Asia (other than China, Japan, and India) ranked third after Europe and has grown quickly. See Justin Chakma et al, "Asia's Ascent—Global Trends in Biomedical R&D Expenditures," *New England Journal of Medicine*, January 2, 2014.

8 Murphy and Topel, "The Economic Value of Medical Research," 7.

9 J. Sanford Schwartz, "Health Services Research: Translating Discovery and Research into Practice and Policy," David Robertson and Gordon H. Williams, eds., *Clinical and Translational Science: Principles of Human Research* (London, England: Elsevier/

Academic Press, 2009), 543ff.

10 Or almost real time. Most famously in the Cuban missile crisis of 1962, when American ambassador to the UN Adlai Stevenson angrily called out his Soviet counterpart about the placement of long range missiles in Cuba: "Just answer the question, yes or no—and you don't have to wait for the translation!"

11 Italo Biaggioni, "Industry-Sponsored Clinical Research in Academia," Robertson and Williams, 184; T. F. Bumol and A. M. Watanabe, "Genetic Information, Genomic Technologies and the Future of Drug Discovery," *Journal of the American Medical Association (JAMA)* 285 (2001), 551ff.

12 G. P. Pisano, *Science Business: The Promise, the Reality and the Future of Biotech* (Boston MA: HBS Press, 2007).

13 G. A. Fitzgerald, "Drugs, Industry and Academia," *Science* 320 (2008).

14 See William F. Crowley, "A Stepwise Approach to a Career in Translational Research," Robertson and Williams, 201ff.

15 Robertson and Williams, *Clinical and Translational Science: Principles of Human Research*, xiii.

16 *Ibid.*, xvii–xviii.

17 E. H. Ahrens, Jr., "The Birth of Patient-Oriented Research as a Science," *Perspectives in Biology and Medicine* 38 (1995), 548–53; also Robertson and Williams, 171ff.

18 E. V. Newman and J. S. Greathouse, Jr., "The Relationship of the Medical School and Hospital to the Clinical Research Center," *Journal of Medical Education* (1963), 38: 514–17; F. C. Luft, "The Role of the General Clinical Research Center in Promoting Patient-oriented Research into the Mechanisms of Disease," *Journal of Molecular Medicine* (1997), 75: 545–50.

19 Robertson and Williams, 173.

20 E. A. Zerhouni, "Translational and Clinical Science—Time for a New Vision," *New England Journal of Medicine* (2005), 353: 1621–23; "Clinical Research at a Crossroads: the NIH Roadmap," *Journal of Investigative Medicine* (2006), 54: 171–73.

21 Robertson and Williams, 174.

22 *Ibid.*, 180.

23 For current assessment, see the 2013 Institute of Medicine report, "The CTSA Program at NIH: Opportunities for Advancing Clinical and Translational Research," www.iom.edu/reports/2013.

24 See https://www.dtmi.duke.edu.

25 See https://www. stsiweb.org.

26 Following, see Donald E. Stokes, *Pasteur's Quadrant: Basic Science and Technological Innovation* (Washington, DC: Brookings Institution Press, 1997), 84.

27 *Ibid.*, 86.

28 *Ibid.*, 87; also see Richard R. Nelson and Sidney G. Winter, *An Evolutionary Theory of Economic Change* (Cambridge, MA: Harvard University Press, 1982).

29 Stokes, *Pasteur's Quadrant: Basic Science and Technological Innovation*, 89.

30 *Ibid.*, 134–35.

31 See National Academy of Sciences, Science, *Technology and the Federal Government: National Goals for a New Era* (Washington, DC: National Academies Press, 1993).

32 It was Pasteur's dictum that "there is no pure science and applied science but only science and the applications of sciences," see Stokes, 106. Starting in 2003, the NIH Roadmap/Common Fund has pushed the principle of transformative research across administrative and disciplinary lines, emphasizing innovative tools and technologies, use of large data sets, and encouraging high-risk/high-reward projects. Projects must be transformative in that they have high potential "to dramatically affect biomedical and/or behavioral research over the next decade," and catalytic in that they must achieve "a defined set of high-impact goals within 5 to 10 years." See http://commonfund.nih.gov; also Francis Collins et al, "NIH Roadmap/Common Fund at 10 Years," *Science* 345: 6194, July 18, 2014.

33 See Figure 26.1, Robertson and Williams, 384.

34 John C. Alexander and Daniel E. Salazar, "Modern Drug Discovery and Development," Robertson and Williams, 361ff.

35 The premise of Pisano, *Science Business*.

36 Christopher H. Colecchi, Roger Kitterman, et al, "Translating Science to the Bedside: The Innovation Pipeline," Robertson and Williams, 383–85.

37 *Ibid.*, 384.

38 *Ibid.*, 389.

39 *Ibid.*, 390.

40 *Ibid.*, 391.

41 *Ibid.*, 396.

42 Following, Jeff Conn, Professor of Pharmacology and Director of Drug Discovery, Vanderbilt University Medical Center, interview with authors, June 23, 2008.

43 Rewards matters, and academe's and industry's are different. Conn: "I can't tell you how many tenure and promotion committee meeting I've been in where someone's denied tenure because they worked too closely with another faculty and you couldn't

tell whether it's really their work." Interview with authors, June 23, 2008.

44 Alexander and Salazar, "Modern Drug Discovery and Development," in Robertson and Williams, 361–76.

45 See www.fda.gov/oc/initiatives/criticalpath.

46 Jeff Conn, interview with authors, June 23, 2008.

47 *Ibid.*

48 Jeff Conn and Lee Limbird, conversation with authors, November 5, 2009.

49 Jeff Conn, interview with authors, June 23, 2008.

50 Abraham Flexner, *I Remember*; Thomas Neville Bonner, *Iconoclast: Abraham Flexner and a Life in Learning*; Timothy C. Jacobson, *Making Medical Doctors: Science and Medicine at Vanderbilt Since Flexner.*

51 The argument here from Pisano, *Science Business*, 191ff.

52 See F. H. Knight, *Risk, Uncertainty and Profit* (Boston, MA: Houghton Mifflin, 1921).

53 Pisano, *Science Business*, 9, 188.

54 *Ibid.*, 12.

55 *Ibid.*, 152–53.

56 *Ibid.*, 13.

57 Pisano, *Science Business*, 3.

58 Association of University Technology Managers (AUTM), *Annual Report*, 2007.

59 Pisano, *Science Business*, 190; Richard R. Nelson, *Technology, Institutions and Economic Growth* (Cambridge, MA: Harvard University Press, 2005).

60 Following, see surveys in Diane Palmintera et al, "Report to the Connecticut Technology Transfer and Commercialization Advisory Board of the Governor's Competitiveness Council," Innovation Associates, Inc., 2004.

61 *Ibid.*, 63–64.

62 *Ibid.*, 66.

63 *Ibid.*, 81–91, regarding Penn.

64 *Ibid.*, 93-102; www.warf.org.

65 *Ibid.*, 97.

66 Other exemplary cases from the Innovation Associates: MIT, Carnegie Mellon University, Washington University, University of California, San Diego, and Cambridge University.

67 *Ibid.*, 130.

Two: Making Truth Useful

1 It is neither. In this book, we split the difference, stipulating a definition of medicine as a science-utilizing practice, focused on individuals and that can have impact on the health of populations. We are indebted here to Kathryn Montgomery, *How Doctors Think: Clinical Judgment and the Practice of Medicine* (New York, NY: Oxford University Press, 2006).

2 See Charles Rosenberg, *Our Present Complaint: American Medicine Then and Now* (Baltimore, MD: Johns Hopkins University Press, 2007), 4–7. Also, Stefan Timmermans and Marc Berg, *The Gold Standard: The Challenge of Evidenced-Based Medicine and Standardization in Health Care* (Philadelphia, PA: Temple University Press, 2003); Jeanne Daley, *Evidence-Based Medicine and the Search for a Science of Clinical Care* (Berkeley, CA: University of California Press, 2005).

3 D. L. Sackett et al, "Evidence-based Medicine: What It Is and What It Isn't," *British Medical Journal,* 312: 71–72 (1996).

4 Timmermans and Berg, *The Gold Standard*, viii.

5 K. Dickersin and E. Manheimer, "The Cochrane Collaboration Evaluation of Health Care and Services Using Systematic Reviews of the Results of Randomized Controlled Trials, *Clinical Obstetrics and Gynecology,* 41: 315–31, 1998.

6 "Evidence-Based Medicine Working Group: Evidence-based medicine: a new approach to teaching the practice of medicine, *Journal of the American Medical Association (JAMA)*, 268: 2420–25, 1992.

7 Sackett et al, 1996.

8 That evidence-based guidelines have been ascribed "gold-standard status" as the measure of good clinical practice does not mean that the standard is fixed. It means that it is universally acknowledged and that its contents are uniformly applied. The content of evidence-base standards evolves with discovery however, and in this respect it trumps its gold-standard inspiration from the world of finance. Tying currencies tightly to gold reserves, as was widely practiced in the nineteenth and twentieth centuries, assured convertibility of financial assets and facilitated trade. Evidence-based guidelines are likewise intended to be recognized everywhere, though their value is likely to increase with discovery over time. See Timmermans and Berg, *The Gold Standard*.

9 David Eddy, "Evidence-Based Medicine: A Unified Approach," *Health Affairs,* 24: 9–17 (January/February 2005).

10 Sackett et al, 2000.

11 Language of Florida State University School of Medicine Evidence-based Tutorial; www.med.fsu.edu/index.cfm.

12 Institute of Medicine, 1992.

13 Wiener; *Chasm* p. 151.

14 Lawrence Weed, "The Computer as a New Basis for Analytical Clinical Practice." *Mt. Sinai Journal of Medicine*, 52: 94–98 (1985).

15 Following see Canadian Institutes of Health; http://ktclearinghouse.ca/cebm.

16 See content.healthaffairs.org/cgi/content/full/hlthaff/24/1/9/DC1.

17 *Ibid.*

18 Cochrane currently lists some two dozen databases and is constantly updating.

19 Following, see *Sense About Science*, cases from the Academy of Medical Royal Colleges UK, April 2013.

20 F. Sullivan, et al, "Early Treatment with Prednisolone or Acyclovir in Bell's Palsy," *New England Journal of Medicine*, 357: 1598–1607 (2007).

21 Patrick F. van Rheenen et al, "Fecal calprotectin for screening of patients with suspected inflammatory bowel disease: diagnostic meta-analysis," *British Medical Journal*, 341:3369 (2010).

22 NICE Guideline on CardioQ-ODM (esophageal Doppler monitor); www. Nice.org. uk/MTG3.

23 Liggins and Howie, "A controlled trial of antepartum glucocorticoid treatment for prevention of respiratory distress syndrome in premature infants," (1972).

24 G. Thorpe-Beeston, "Outcome of breech delivery at term," *British Medical Journal*, 305: 746–7 (1992).

25 "Standardization of Breast Radiotherapy 2008 Trial A of radiotherapy hypofractionation for treatment of early breast cancer: randomized trial," *Lancet Oncology*, 9: 331–41.

26 M A. Fischl, D. D. Richmond, M. H. Grieco, et al "The Efficacy of azidothymidine (AZT) in the treatment of patients with AIDS and AIDS-related complex. A double-blind, placebo-controlled trial," *New England Journal of Medicine*, 317: 185 (1987); Panel on treatment of HIV-infested pregnant women and prevention of perinatal transmission, Department of Health and Human Services, 2010, at aidsinfo.nih.gov/Content Files/PerinatalGL.pdf.

27 B. Damato and S. E. Coupland, "Translating uveal melanoma cytogenetics into clinical care," *Archives of Ophthalmology*, 127: 423029 (2009).

28 C. A. Jackevicius, P. Li, J. V. Tu, "Prevalence, predictors, and outcomes of primary nonadherence after acute myocardial infarction," *Circulation,* 117: 1028–36 (2008).

29 David L. Sackett, et al, "Evidence based medicine: what it is and what it isn't," *British Medical Journal,* 71–72.

30 See "Evidence-based Medicine in its place," *Lancet,* 346: 785 (1995); recounted in Richard Smith and Drummond Rennie, "Evidence-based Medicine—And Oral History," *Journal of the American Medical Association (JAMA)* 311: 365–67 (2014).

31 Sackett in Daley, *Evidence-Based Medicine and the Search for a Science of Clinical Care,* 1.

32 See Trisha Greenhalgh, "Narrative based medicine in an evidence based world," *British Medical Journal,* 318: 323 (1999).

33 http://www.qmul.ac.uk/media/news/items/smd/134739.html.

34 For example, Florian Naudet and Bruno Falissard, "Does reduction ad absurdum have a place in evidence-based medicine?" *BioMed Central Medicine* 12: 106 (2014): "The story told by an RCT [randomized control trial] focuses on efficacy, sometimes effectiveness, and specifically on the pre-post difference in a very limited aspect of the average patient. This story does not tell much about the individual patient's story that a clinician is fact with and ignores an entire segment of therapeutics that plays a crucial role: care that draws on what we might call the patient's 'irrationality,' which has no place in mainstream evidence-based stories."

35 Using an example of nonvalvular atrial fibrillation in a patient with small risk of stroke, EBM founder and epidemiologist David Sackett illustrated how EBM must meld research evidence with clinical skills with patient values and experiences. He asked: "Should the patient take warfarin and so risk a bleed?" And he answered: "Most patients see a stroke as about 4 times worse than a bleed. You combine that with number needed to treat and number needed to harm and conclude that you are about 11 times more likely to help rather than harm a patient by treating him with warfarin." "Evidence-Based Medicine: An Oral History," 366.

Three: Teams Work

1 See Paul Starr, *The Social Transformation of American Medicine: The Rise of a Sovereign Profession and the Making of a Vast Industry* (New York, NY: Basic, 1984).

2 See John R. Katzenbach and Douglas K. Smith, *The Wisdom of Teams: Creating the High-Performance Organization* (New York, NY: HarperCollins, 1993), *passim.*

3 This educational deficit, while still deep, is not unrecognized. See Molly Cooke, et al *Educating Physicians: A Call for Reform of Medical School and Residency* (Carnegie Foundation for the Advancement of Teaching, 2010).

4 See David Lawrence, *From Chaos to Care: the Promise of Team-Based Medicine* (Cambridge, MA: Perseus, 2002); the equivalent for health care of *The Wisdom of Teams*.

5 Following, David Lawrence, interview with authors, January 22, 2010.

6 *Ibid.*

7 See Thomas A. Kochan et al, *Healing Together: The Labor-Management Partnership at Kaiser Permanente* (Ithaca, NY: Cornell University Press, 2009).

8 Lawrence, *From Chaos to Care.*

9 That report, much reported at the time (2001), invited disappointment in its very subtitle, "A New Health System for the 21st Century." What once had been mere "medicine," thence "health care," became here nothing less than "health" itself (although, of coursem undefined). See Institute of Medicine, *Crossing the Quality Chasm: A New Health System for the 21st Century*, 2001.

10 J. D. Kleinke, *Oxymorons: The Myth of the US Health Care System* (San Francisco, CA, 2001).

11 Lawrence, *From Chaos to Care*, 133ff.

12 New in the sense that still a minority of medical professionals emerges from their education systematically trained in teamwork and working collaboratively.

13 Lawrence, *From Chaos to Care*, 133ff; Norman Gevitz, *The DOs: Osteopathic Medicine in America* (Baltimore, MD: Johns Hopkins University Press, 2004).

14 Lawrence, *From Chaos to Care*, 145.

15 The Asthma Sinus Allergy Program at Vanderbilt University Medical Center ("ASAP").

16 Simpson B. Tanner, interview with authors, February 11, 2010.

17 *Ibid.*

18 *Ibid.*

19 Susan Ficken, interview with authors, February 12, 2010.

20 *Ibid.*

21 ASAP ran through more than half a dozen different administrators in its first five or six years.

22 Vanderbilt Heart and Vascular Institute.

23 Keith and Andre Churchwell, interviews with authors, February 12, 2010.

24 And thus the massive "clinical enterprise" in contemporary AHCs, a reality that

Flexner (who aimed at all costs to insulate academic medicine from the market: thus "full-time") would have found abhorrent.

25 Churchwell interviews.

26 *Ibid.*

27 See Lucian Leape Institute white paper, "Unmet Needs: Teaching Physicians to Provide Safe Patient Care," October 2009.

28 David Lawrence, interview with authors, January 2010.

29 See Clayton Christiansen, Jerome Grossman, and Jason Hwang, *The Innovator's Prescription: A Disruptive Solution for Health Care* (New York, NY: McGraw-Hill, 2009).

30 David Lawrence, interview with authors, November 5, 2009.

Four: Informatics Order

1 Or almost right. Osler thought bleeding sound practice.

2 Daniel Masys interview with authors, April 1, 2009. Some argue even that biology, like chemistry (née alchemy) before it, is set to become "a predictable, repeatable science" and that what was formerly a discovery science is now an information science. Menno Prins (Philips Electronics) and Ajay Royyuru (IBM), *Economist*, April 18, 2009. Also, Michael Fourman, "Informatics," Division of Informatics Centre for Intelligent Systems and their Application, University of Edinburgh, Informatics Research Report; http://www.informatics.ed.ac.uk/.

3 See Leiyu Shi and Douglas A. Singh, *Delivering Health Care in America: A Systems Approach* (Boston, MA: Jones and Bartlett, 2008).

4 Daniel Masys, interview with authors, April 1, 2009.

5 A 2005 RAND Corporation report on digitization of health systems forecast savings of $77 billion a year if 90 percent of doctors and hospitals were to implement digitized systems. Health and safety benefits would push the figure even higher. Also see Annals of Internal Medicine study, January 2009.

6 Following, "Strategic Plan for Informatics and Roadmap to 2010," Vanderbilt Department of Informatics, 2005.

7 America's largest single provider of integrated care, Kaiser Permanente, testifies to both improved efficiency and better outcomes. See *Health Affairs*, March 2009.

8 See Chapter 6, below.

9 Following, William W. Stead, "Electronic Health Records," in Dennis Cortese and

William B. Rouse, eds., *Engineering the System of Health Care Delivery* (Amsterdam, The Netherlands: IOS Press, 2010), 119–144.

10 In 2009, the *New England Journal of Medicine* reported that only 1.5 percent of 3,049 hospitals surveyed had comprehensive electronic records management systems in place. A. K. Jha, C. M. Desroches, et al, "Use of electronic records in US hospitals," Special Article, *New England Journal of Medicine*, March 25, 2009.

11 See William W. Stead and Herbert S. Lin, eds., *Computational Technology for Effective Health Care* (Washington, DC: National Research Council/National Academies Press, 2009).

12 *Crossing the Quality Chasm* (Washington: National Academies Press, 2001).

13 On early development of the electronic medical record, pioneered at Duke University Medical Center in the 1970s, see W. E. Hammond and W. W. Stead, "The Evolution of GEMISCH ["Generalized MIS for Community Health Programming Language"] and TMR ["The Medical Record"]," in H. F. Orthner et al eds., *Implementing Health Care Information Systems* (New York, NY: Springer, 1989), 33–66.

14 Thirty years ago, diabetes mellitus was classified into two types: juvenile onset diabetes and insulin dependent diabetes, one; and adult onset diabetes and non-insulin dependent diabetes, the other. Current knowledge re-classifies things: Type 1 diabetes (autoimmune destruction of insulin-producing beta cells), and Type 2 diabetes (insulin resistance). Both Type 1 and Type 2 however can afflict children or adults, while Type 2 can be insulin-dependent or not.

15 W. W. Stead, "Electronic Health Records," William W. Stead interviews with the authors, September 16, 2008 and June 18, 2009.

16 Daniel Masys, interview with authors, April 1, 2009.

17 Following see M. E. Frisse et al, "A regional health information exchange: architecture and implementation," *American Medical Informatics Symposium Proceedings*, 2008, 212–218.

18 Roden, et al.

19 Stead and J. M. Starmer, "Beyond Expert-based practice," IOM Annual Meeting Summary, 2008.

20 Daniel Masys, interview with authors, April 1, 2009.

21 *Ibid.*

22 *Ibid.*

23 See *Health Affairs*, March 2009.

Five: Ever Better

1 Peter Drucker, *The Concept of the Corporation* (New York, NY: John Day, 1946).

2 Following, see summary in James P. Womack, Daniel T. Jones and Daniel Roos, *The Machine that Changed the World: The Story of Lean Production, How Japan's Secret Weapon in the Global Auto Wars Will Revolutionize Western Industry* (New York, NY: Free Press, 1990).

3 Gary Kaplan, interview with authors, October 26, 2009.

4 The full story: Charles Kenney, *Transforming Health Care: Virginia Mason Medical Center's Pursuit of the Perfect Patient Experience* (New York, NY: Productivity Press, 2010).

5 *Ibid.*, also Charles Kenney, *The Best Practice* (New York, NY: Public Affairs, 2008), 161 ff.

6 Gary Kaplan, interview with authors, October 26, 2009.

7 The central text is John Black, *A World Class Production System* (Boeing, 1998); also Mary Walton and W. Edwards Deming,The Deming Management Method (New York, NY: Dodd Mead, 1986).

8 Following, Gary S. Kaplan, MD, "Seeking Perfection in Health Care: Applying the Toyota Production System to Medicine," Virginia Mason Center for Corporate Innovation, 2008.

9 *Ibid.*

10 *Ibid.*

11 Value-added defined as "part of the process that changes the form, fit or function of the product or service, and something that the customer is willing to pay for." Non value-added inserts "not" between is and willing.

12 The only public national comparison of hospitals on key issues such as mortality rates for key common procedures, infection rates, safety practices and measures of efficiency.

13 Kaplan, "Seeking Perfection in Health Care."

14 *Ibid.*

15 Gary Kaplan, interview with authors, October 26, 2009.

16 A. J. Cronin, *The Citadel* (London, England: Gollancz, 1937). Cronin was both novelist and doctor.

17 Kenney, *The Best Practice*, 176.

18 Gary Kaplan, interview with authors, October 26, 2009.

19 www.geisinger.edu.

20 *Ibid.*

21 Glenn J. Steele testimony to Senate Committee on Finance, "Reforming the Health care Delivery System," April 21, 2009.

22 R. Abelson, "In a Bid for Better Care: Surgery with a Warranty," *New York Times*, May 17, 2007.

23 *Ibid.*

24 See A. Casale, et al, "A Provider-Driven Pay-for-Performance Program for Acute Episodic Cardiac Surgical Care," *Annals of Surgery*, October 2007.

25 Steele testimony to Senate Committee on Finance, April 21, 2009; http://www.geisinger.org/provencare/as_pdf.

26 *Ibid.*

27 The founding story of the IHI is well-told in Kenney, *The Best Practice*, 39ff.

28 *Ibid.*, 55.

29 See Quint Studer, *Hardwiring Excellence: Purpose, Worthwhile Work, Making a Difference* (Gulf Breeze, Florida, 2003).

30 Studer called these "values," though "needs" is more precise; people respond to needs but hold values.

31 Studer, *Hardwiring Excellence*, 29.

32 The work of renowned book designer Gary Gore, the medical center's three-circling arrows logo—for research, teaching and patient care, with a bold V at the center—was a classic of graphic clarity that proved exceptionally durable, serving from the 1970s until 2010 when the medical center brand was subsumed into that of the university.

33 Studer used the example of one hospital that predicted that it could add $2 million to its bottom line for each point reduction in employee turnover.

34 The nine: Commit to Excellence, Measure the Important Things, Build a Culture Around Service, Create and Develop Leaders, Focus on Employee Satisfaction, Build Individual Accountability, Align Behavior with Goals and Values, Communicate at All Levels, Recognize and Reward Success.

35 W. Edwards Deming, Foreword to Mary Walton, *Deming Management at Work* (New York, NY: Putnam, 1990), 10.

36 W. Edwards Deming, "Notes on Management in a Hospital," September 20, 1987; see *Ibid.*, 84.

37 Studer interview with authors October 28, 2009.

Six: 1919: Getting It Done Now

1 An example of one such "only-the-will-is-lacking" admonition: Molly Cooke, David Irby et al, "American Medical Education 100 Years After the Flexner Report," *New England Journal of Medicine*, September 28, 2006.

2 *The Flexner Report*, 20.

3 Today, there are fewer but more highly regulated schools, 141, enrolling more students, 82,000, to serve a population of 317 million.

4 For a highly original "epidemiological" analysis of the impact of the *Flexner Report* on school closings, see Mark D. Hiatt and Christopher Stockton, "The Impact of the Flexner Report on the Fate of Medical Schools in North America After 1909," *Journal of American Physicians and Surgeons* (2003) 8: 37–40. The authors conclude that probably 20+ percent of the 168 schools (including Canadian ones) closed as a direct result of a bad grade from Flexner. To determine whether an "environmental factor" is the cause of a disease (the analogue "environmental factor" here being the Report, the "disease" the closing of a school), they used a set of criteria originated by British statistician Austin Bradford Hill and which, they asserted the Report satisfied: "temporality (Flexner's inspections preceded the rash of closings and mergers in subsequent years); dose-response (the casualty list of schools contains a high proportion of the ones most harshly criticized); consistency (many researchers have placed Flexner at the root of the reduction in the number of schools); plausibility (disfavored schools subsequently found it difficult to secure funding from foundations and governments and licensure for their students from state regulatory boards); and analogy (similar surveys have had a similar effect.)"

5 Bonner, *Iconoclast*, 69.

6 See Steven C. Wheatley, *The Politics of Philanthropy: Abraham Flexner and Medical Education* (Madison, WI: University of Wisconsin Press, 1988), 140–41.

7 Abraham Flexner, "Medical Education in the United States: A Program," June 1919, Abraham Flexner Papers, Box 11, Library of Congress.

8 The distributed list: New England: Harvard and Yale (2); Middle and Atlantic: "universities in New York, Philadelphia, Pittsburgh, Baltimore, Syracuse or Rochester and Howard University at Washington (6); North Central: "at Cincinnati, Columbus, Cleveland, Chicago, Indianapolis (5); Middle West and West: "Minneapolis, Iowa City, St. Louis, Kansas City, Omaha, Denver, Salt Lake City, San Francisco, Seattle, Portland (12); South: see below (6). *Ibid.*

9 Bonner, *Iconoclast*, 146ff.

10 "Medical Education in the United States: A Program," June 1919, Flexner Papers.

11 Abraham Flexner, "Memorandum Regarding Mr. Rockefeller's Gift to be Devoted to the Improvement of Medical Education in the United Stated," December 1919, Abraham Flexner Papers, Box 11, Library of Congress.

12 "Medical Education in the United States: A Program," June 1919, Flexner Papers.

13 *Ibid.*

14 Bonner, *Iconoclast*, 172.

15 Wheatley, *The Politics of Philanthropy*, ix.

16 Bonner, *Iconoclast*, 170.

17 Bonner, *Iconoclast*, 162; Jacobson, *Making Medical Doctors*, 81ff.

18 Elizabeth Brayer, *George Eastman: A Biography* (Rochester, NY: University of Rochester Press, 2012).

19 *Educating Physicians: A Call for Reform of Medical School and Residency* (San Francisco, CA: Jossey-Bass, 2010).

20 "A mini-version of the Flexner initiative," was how one observer described it. See Thomas P. Duffy, "The Flexner Report 100 Years Later," *Yale Journal of Biology and Medicine* (2011) 84: 269–76. The chosen fourteen: Atlantic Health, Morristown, New Jersey; Cambridge Hospital, Cambridge, Massachusetts; Henry Ford Hospital and Medical Center, Detroit; Northwestern University; Mayo Medical Center; Southern Illinois University; University of California, San Francisco; University of Florida, Gainesville and Jacksonville; University of Minnesota; University of North Dakota; University of Pennsylvania; University of South Florida, Tampa, University of Texas Medical Branch, Galveston; University of Washington, Seattle.

21 *Ibid.*; also David Irby, "Educating Physicians for the Future: Carnegie's Calls for Reform," *Medical Teacher* 33: 547–550 (2011).

22 On the popularly accepted proposition that health care and even health are positive rights, see in summary Jonathan Wolff, *The Human Right to Health* (New York, NY: W. W. Norton & Company, Inc., 2012). On the argument that no such rights exists and that positing them had led into hopeless policy quagmires, see Richard A. Epstein, *Mortal Peril: Our Inalienable Right to Health Care?* (Cambridge, MA: Perseus, 1999); Alasdair MacIntyre, *After Virtue: A Study in Moral Theory* (Notre Dame, IN: University of Notre Dame Press, second edition, 1984), 69–70; Bernard A. Baumrin, "Why There Is No Right To Health Care," in Rosamond Rhodes et al, eds., *Medicine and Social Justice: Essays on the Distribution of Health Care* (New York,

NY: Oxford University Press, 2002), 78–83.

23 This concept of viewing health-care delivery as a collection of demand modules was shared in interviews with the authors by David Lawrence, former CEO of Kaiser Permanente, January 22, 2010.

24 See Elizabeth A. McGlynn et al, "The Quality of Health Care Delivered to Adults in the United States," New England Journal of Medicine 348: 2635-2645 (June 26, 2003)

25 Cheryl Damberg et al, *Measuring Success in Health Care Value-based Purchasing Programs: Summary and Recommendations* (Santa Monica, CA: Rand Corporation, 2014).

26 Other philanthropists before long joined the parade, so that over the next two decades total philanthropic commitment to Flexner's program went to the hundreds of millions.

27 See John A. Spertus, "Leveraging Entrepreneurship as a Means to Improve the Translation of Outcomes Research to Healthcare Improvement"; http://circoutcomes. ahajournals.org. Accessed January 20, 2015.

28 Bonner, *Iconoclast*, 170.

CPSIA information can be obtained
at www.ICGtesting.com
Printed in the USA
BVHW04*1146300518
517730BV00007B/49/P